D0514498

WHO'S NEXT?

Books available from the same author

By Appointment Only series:
Arthritis, Rheumatism and Psoriasis (5th impression)
Asthma and Bronchitis
Cancer and Leukemia (2nd impression)
Heart and Blood Circulatory Problems
Life Without Arthritis – The Maori Way
Migraine and Epilepsy (3rd impresion)
The Miracle of Life (2nd impression)
Multiple Sclerosis (4th impression)
Neck and Back Problems (4th impression)
Realistic Weight Control (2nd impression)
Skin Diseases
Stress and Nervous Disorders (3rd impression)
Traditional Home and Herbal Remedies (5th impression)
Viruses, Allergies and the Immune System (4th impression)

Nature's Gift series:
Body Energy (2nd impression)
Water – Healer or Poison?
Food

Well Woman series:
Menstual and Pre-menstrual Tension

WHO'S NEXT?

JAN DE VRIES

*The
Humorous
Reminiscences
of an Alternative
Medical Practitioner*

Illustrations by PETER FOYLE

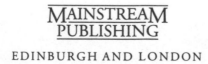

MAINSTREAM
PUBLISHING

EDINBURGH AND LONDON

This edition 1993
First published in 1989 by
MAINSTREAM PUBLISHING CO. (EDINBURGH) LTD
7 Albany Street
Edinburgh EH1 3UG

ISBN 1 85158 516 8

A catalogue record for this book is available from the British Library

Typeset in Palatino
Reproduced from disc by Polyprint, Edinburgh
Printed and bound in Great Britain by BPCC Wheatons, Exeter

The names of characters in this book and certain events described therein have been altered to avoid any possible embarrassment to the individuals concerned.

Contents

Alternative Medicine Man

Gin ye should spiflicate yer spine
And yints are jerkit oot o' line,
Frae pain, alas, there's nae release,
Until ye gang tae Jan de Vries.

Ye suffer torture in yer kyte,
For weeks yer in an awfu plight;
And scunnert, noo, wi castor ile,
It's tlme ye gaed tae Auchenkyle.

Yer girth is forty inches roon,
Yer wecht, ye canna get it doon;
And ten tae wan it will increase,
Unless ye gang tae Jan de Vries.

Ye hae arthritis in yer banes
And walkin racks ye, fu' o' pains;
But skeich ye'd be tae rin a mile,
Gin ye wad gang tae Auchenkyle.

Gin ye're afflictit unco sair
And doakters dinna help nae mair,
Yer aches and pains will a' decrease,
When in the hauns o' Jan de Vries.

Ye've smokit fags for mony a year,
The consequences, noo, ye fear;
Ye needna swither for a while,
It's time ye rung up Auchenkyle.

It's faur ower late tae hope and pray;
Get on the phone withoot delay!
When contemplatin yer decease,
Yer only hope is Jan de Vries!

John Boyd (a patient)

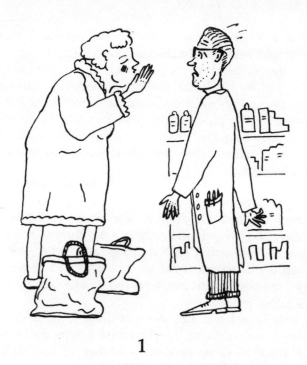

1

Her Fatal Attraction

WEEK IN, WEEK out, she used to come into town on her old bike and at the end of her shopping trip she would call into the pharmacy. The two bags hanging on either side of the luggage carrier of her bike would be loaded to overflowing with provisions. She would always arrive at our pharmacy at lunch-time. Her name was Mrs Clean, although this in itself was a laugh, as she did not do her name justice. By anyone's standards she was far from clean and, dare I say it, she was also far from attractive.

Every week she called into the pharmacy for the same errand and it was usually me who was sent down to serve her. Our pharmacy was in a very old building in a lovely old town in the Netherlands. The stock-room was on a different level to the shop itself. For obvious reasons, the dispensary bordered the stock-rooms. Let us not forget that in those days most prescriptions had to be individually prepared by the pharmacist; powders had to be mixed and pills were handmade. Few medicines were available ready-made on demand from the pharmaceutical manufacturers or wholesalers.

When there were no customers in the shop, the staff would usually be busy upstairs helping out. Whenever a customer opened the door to the shop, a bell would ring and someone would make their way down. We could see what was happening in the shop and who was entering through a plate-glass window . . . and as I remember it, it always seemed to be me who was sent down when Mrs Clean called in.

At that time I was not yet qualified. I could handle most counter sales as these rarely caused any problems, but I could always call in another member of the staff if I did encounter any difficulty. As Mrs Clean always made the same purchase, she was an easy customer.

On this occasion, however, after I had served her as usual, Mrs Clean took her time and looked around before starting to leave the premises. Then she came back to the counter. Self-consciously she approached me with the words: "Could I ask you for some personal advice?"

Although greatly taken aback, of course I assured her that I would try to be of help. Please remember that I was still very young and inexperienced. I was therefore flabbergasted when I heard her question. If only I had had the sense to call another member of staff at that point, but no such luck!

She proceeded to tell me that her husband was considerably older than herself and that they had several children. However, every day after supper her husband felt amorous and wanted to retire with her. She blushed while telling me that she had become less and less inclined to give in to his amorous demands and therefore it appeared that she was unable to perform to his expectations. I tried to cover up my embarrassment by appearing to think deeply on the matter but, as if this were a request for further information, she continued by supplying me with even more personal details.

By now shivers were running up and down my spine and I decided, there and then, that I never wanted to have anything whatsoever to do with sex. Suffice to say, that one is entitled to change one's mind when growing up!

However, the big question remained: how on earth was I going to answer her? By that time I felt definitely too entangled to nip up the stairs and involve any of the other staff. I imagine that it would usually have been my aunt, who was the pharmacist, who would deal with any questions in this field, but things had gone too far for me to go and call her down. I would have had to give her an explanation and even the thought of doing so made me feel embarrassed. I then decided to take the bull by the horns and suggested that Mrs Clean purchase some tranquillisers for her husband.

When Mrs Clean informed me that he would never willingly agree to take a tranquillising tablet, I went further and suggested that she administer it surreptitiously. How about pulverising a tablet and adding it to his porridge?

She duly purchased a bottle of tranquillisers and left the premises. Whatever happened after that is anyone's guess, but I never saw Mrs Clean again. My colleagues often wondered what might have happened to her, as she had been such a regular customer for so long — once a week at lunchtime. Believe me, I never let on about what I considered at one time to have been a most delicate situation!

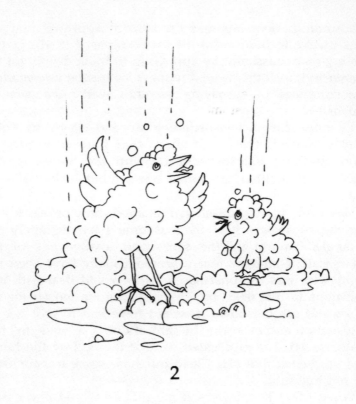

2

Bird Brains

ONE DAY, two little boys came up to the counter in the pharmacy where I was doing my apprenticeship. I knew them as the two young sons of a well-to-do local gentleman farmer. Timidly, they asked me for something with which to wash the sparrows' hair. I thought that I must have misunderstood what they meant and therefore asked them to repeat themselves. Still none the wiser, I explained to them that nature takes care of that and sparrows do not need to be washed as rainwater does this quite effectively. I also explained that sparrows have feathers, not hair.

"Our sparrows have hair," insisted the older of the pair.

A grubby hand was placed on the counter to show me some money and they again told me that their mother had been insistent they come back with something with which to wash the sparrows' hair. I could hear one or two of the other customers sniggering in the background, but the boys stood their ground and I was beginning to feel sorry for them. If it had been another time of the year, I would have thought that they had been sent out on a wild goose chase, because to me it sounded like an April Fool's joke.

I decided to telephone their mother for clarification so that she could tell me herself what she wanted and save the lads a second journey. When I asked them for their name and telephone number, I immediately realised that a telephone call was superfluous. Their mother had indeed sent them for something for the sparrows' hair. What they wanted was shampoo and their name was Sparrow!

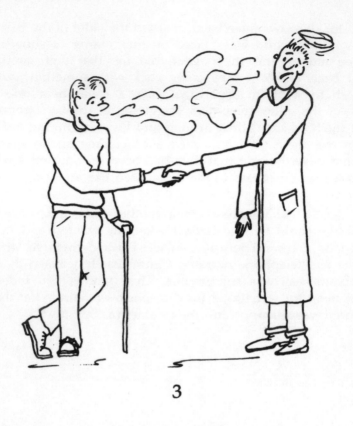

3

Mind over Matter

AT THE PHARMACY where I worked during my years of study, I was consulted by an elderly gentleman. He told me that he had great difficulty walking and was lucky if he could manage a few hundred yards at a time. On the whole, considering his age, he was still quite fit and healthy and had plenty of energy. He explained that if it had not been for his legs, he would be able to get out and enjoy himself. He desperately wanted to be able to go and visit his friends, instead of having to sit at home and wait for them to call in on him.

Just about that time the newspapers were giving a great deal of publicity to the beneficial properties of garlic and this herb had recently become available on the market in tablet form. This very simple remedy — still greatly valued today by many regular users — had been the subject of numerous "miracle" stories in the press, with the most remarkable recoveries being accredited to the use of garlic tablets.

We discussed this trend and some of the claims that had been made and the elderly gentleman asked me if I knew personally of anyone who had used the remedy successfully. Unfortunately I did not, but nevertheless he decided to give it a try.

Three weeks later he reappeared in the shop to purchase a further supply of garlic tablets and I remarked upon the fact that he looked particularly lively. He proudly informed me that he had increased his intake to six garlic tablets per day. He had never felt better and his walking had improved beyond imagination. He added that, apart from losing most of his friends, he was now the happiest man in the world. Anyway, he was now able to call on his friends and they would soon get used to the particular aroma that enveloped him!

This experience proves, as I have witnessed so often over the years, how the power of fervent desire combined with the psychology of whole-hearted conviction can eventually bear fruit.

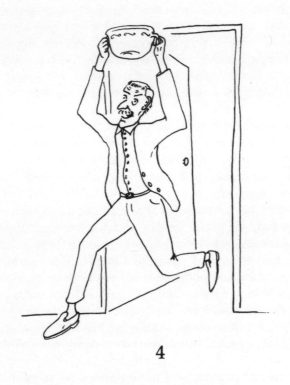

4

Willing to Share

AFTER I GRADUATED as a pharmacist, my life changed direction drastically. Shortly after I had finished my pharmaceutical studies, I decided to diversify into alternative medicine. Later, when I had qualified for my studies in homoeopathy, naturopathy and osteopathy, the well-known Swiss naturopath Dr Alfred Vogel invited me to open the first clinic for alternative therapies in the Netherlands.

My time at this well-organised clinic has left me with countless memories. Thinking back to those early days, disconcerting and humorous memories alike spring easily to mind. Obviously we had our share of seriously ill patients, but we also had our share of malingerers. This may sound unkind and is certainly not meant in an unpleasant manner, but we all know the type of person who is intent on sharing his or her discomfort with others and expects endless sympathy. It is equally true that there are many people who prefer to suffer in silence and from whom we will rarely hear a complaint.

I well remember one of our very first patients who fell into the category of those who insist on sharing their discomfort. He was an elderly gentleman with beautiful, distinguished-looking white hair, who needed treatment to improve his general health. However, he soon became somewhat of a nuisance to his fellow patients, as he insisted on telling everyone how ill he really was. He demanded everyone's attention and sympathy. This was all the more ludicrous, as many of the patients he was surrounded by were much more seriously ill than he.

I spent a fair amount of time with this gentleman and tactfully tried to point out to him that people are rarely interested in someone else's medical history and even if they do listen politely, it is quite enough to hear the story once. In any case, I told him, apart from kidney stones, there was basically very little wrong with him. This he had refused to accept and I already knew that he had previously gone from one source to another in his obsession to get "well" again.

At our clinic it was decided to use an old-fashioned remedy to encourage his body to pass the kidney stones, rather than have him finally having to resort to surgery.

It should be understood that alternative medicine does not have a radical stance *against* surgery. Under certain circumstances surgery seems to be the only answer, but so often surgical operations are performed where alternative medicine can be used successfully in its place. Much money can be saved by avoiding the expense of both the operation itself and the resulting need for a lengthy period of convalescence in hospital. Moreover, the traumatic shock to the patient's system is considerably minimised by the gentler methods of alternative medicine.

This particular, very concerned patient had developed the habit of studiously examining the results of his bowel and bladder movements, and to facilitate this effort he had accustomed himself to using a chamberpot. One lunchtime he excused himself rather hurriedly from the dining room and returned shortly afterwards proudly carrying his chamberpot.

Greatly excited, he clearly intended to show the contents of this receptacle to his fellow patients, so that they could all share in his delight at seeing there the gritty residue of his kidney stones. Needless to say, one of the medical attendants immediately stepped in to distract our elderly patient, duly fawned over the contents of the chamberpot, and led him sharply out of the dining room before he could upset any of his fellow patients and make a complete fool of himself!

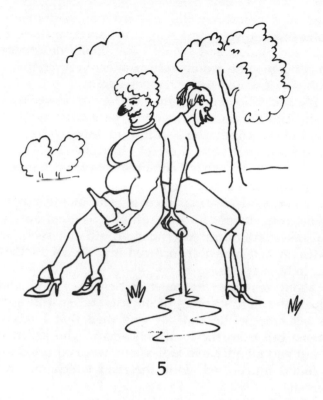

5

Irresistible Temptation

ANOTHER PATIENT in the same residential clinic in the Netherlands comes to mind, whose elephantine size was certainly very apt, as her name, loosely translated, was Mrs Oliphant. She had come to our clinic to lose weight. As the wife of a high-ranking army officer, she had become accustomed to the best of food and drink, as she regularly had to accompany her husband to official functions.

We therefore had a great struggle to keep her on a strict dietary regime and she needed constant supervision. She was very keen to lose weight and tried to co-operate, but only up to a point! We did not attempt to imprison our patients, and in the evening she would sometimes be unable to resist temptation and would occasionally disappear and go on a binge. She would return later, very contrite, and promise that it would never happen again.

During our talks she admitted to having a weakness for chocolate and so we kept a very close eye on her. After a fortnight at the clinic, she had lost an encouraging amount of weight and felt very cheerful about her achievements. Then one afternoon, when I enquired about her, the sister-in-charge informed me that she had gone out to see something of the countryside accompanied by one of the nurses. As the clinic was situated in a beautifully wooded area and it was a glorious autumn afternoon, it did not seem such a bad idea. A taxi had been ordered and the two ladies had set out in high spirits.

By about tea-time, however, when they had still not returned, the first stirrings of unease and suspicion began to be felt among the staff. It was then that I received a telephone call from the local policeman, who asked me to drive out and identify two ladies who were reported to have been found intoxicated along the road which ran through the forest.

When the policeman had picked up the ladies and interviewed them, the only information they had been able to give him in their advanced state of intoxication was the name of our clinic. Needless to say, the ladies proved to be our Mrs Oliphant and the young nurse. I must admit that there had been very little doubt in my mind when I had first heard the policeman's description.

On seeing me, Mrs Oliphant still had the sense to mutter that it had been "only one too many". Both ladies were taken back to the clinic and, no doubt as a result of her deep embarrassment, Mrs Oliphant departed first thing the following morning. This left us with the unenviable task of having to dismiss the nurse who had accompanied her on their escapade, as she had proved herself to be untrustworthy.

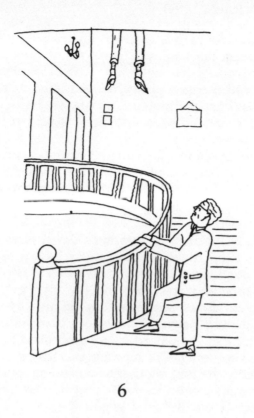

6

Eccentricity to a Tee

AMONG THE STAFF in the clinic in the Netherlands we counted a somewhat unusual character. He was a doctor, highly qualified in orthodox medicine, whose father and grandfather had been eminent medical pioneers. Partly because of his orthodox background, but mostly because of his unusual attitude, he was unsuitable for dealing directly with patients. Nevertheless, he was an excellent researcher and he had been employed largely for that purpose. Only very occasionally was he called upon for night duty, when circumstances were such that we were short of medically qualified staff able to deal with emergencies.

Dr X, as I will call him, was a very tall, gangly person and extremely eccentric. However, the extent of this eccentricity seemed to increase gradually and none of us worried unduly about him, the more so because we had grown used to his whims and oddities and he was seldom in contact with the patients.

One lunch-time, my wife phoned me and, as an aside, she mentioned that Dr X had phoned her earlier and invited himself to pop in for a cup of tea during the afternoon. Apparently, he intended to take a brisk walk through the forest and meant to call on her as he passed the house. As it was a beautiful frosty winter's day, I envied him the opportunity to spare the time for such a long walk.

Shortly afterwards, I saw him walking down the drive from the clinic and could not believe my eyes. There he was, in the middle of winter, setting off on a five-mile walk dressed in a short-sleeved shirt, shorts, sandals and, to top it all, a pith helmet. I ran after him and asked him what he thought he was doing. Did he want to catch pneumonia?

Offhandedly, he told me that he was going for a long walk and had arranged with my wife that he was going to call in for a cup of tea. When I enquired as to the suitability of his mode of dress for the prevailing weather conditions, he politely informed me that it would do his circulation a world of good, and off he marched.

Afterwards, my neighbour told me that he had kept an eye on my wife on seeing this apparition arrive on our doorstep. However, from my wife's greeting when she had opened the door to this odd visitor, my neighbour had realised that she was well acquainted with him and, furthermore, when she had invited him in he had refused and remained outside on the terrace. This helped to set my neighbour's mind at ease, but he had remained alert as to what was happening in our garden and by all accounts he had spent an hilarious afternoon as a spectator.

My wife also told me that my colleague had refused to come in when she answered the door and that he had suggested that they have a cup of tea outside on the terrace. Not having been able to persuade him to change his mind, she had donned a warm coat and joined him briefly out on the terrace. After their cup of tea, she had made her apologies and he had left in good spirits to start on the five-mile walk back to the clinic. She was quite aware of how ludicrous the whole situation must have looked to any occasional passer-by, and felt quite relieved that they had not been spotted by anyone she knew.

When Dr X returned to the clinic he told me that he felt marvellous and even though he had walked about ten miles in total he still intended doing his evening exercises later. Tomorrow he would feel on top of the world!

That evening, at about ten o'clock, our peace at home was rudely disturbed by a telephone call from the clinic. The sister on night duty sounded barely coherent as she begged me to come to the clinic immediately. When I asked her to calm down and explain why I should do so, she told me that Dr X had done himself in. Without further ado I grabbed my coat to leave for the clinic post-haste.

It had to happen on that of all nights: the severe frost had played havoc with my car and, try as I might, I could not get it started. The only way I was going to get to the clinic was to grab a bicycle and pedal as fast as I could. As I cycled in the bitter cold, I began to realise the repercussions this could have on the reputation of the clinic; obviously, too, I was feeling extremely distressed for Dr X.

What could have driven him to commit such an act of desperation? Had we misinterpreted any indications or signals from him? Had he emitted any signals at all, which we had failed to receive?

As is usual with most bystanders under such circumstances, I felt filled with remorse by the time I arrived at the clinic. I should have spent more time with him — and now it was too late.

The sister who had telephoned me met me at the entrance and I followed her silently into the hall, where she stopped and pointed up to the stairwell. There, for all to see, was the dangling body of Dr X, suspended from a rope. His gangly legs seemed even longer than usual, as his trousers had ridden up revealing part of his skinny ankles and calves.

I slowly climbed the stairs and on the third landing I stopped and muttered to myself: "Goodness me Dr X, what on earth drove you to do this?"

The sister, who had followed me up the stairs, turned to me and we stared at each other in stupefaction as we heard Dr X's polished voice: "Good evening, colleague. What brings you back at this time of night?"

The two of us continued to stand and stare for a few moments before we jumped into action. Once we had helped my colleague safely down, he explained to me that he had only been doing his evening exercises. In ignorant bliss of the pandemonium he had caused among the staff, he had been engrossed in meditation.

During our subsequent talk, I pointed out what the implications of such dangerous exercises could be. He lowered his mask slightly and admitted that he was aware that he had been taking things to an extreme. Looking around his room I could well believe that, as I counted at least ten sets of weighing scales. Remarking upon this, he explained that each day it took him an inordinate amount of time to separately weigh his intake of proteins and carboyhdrates. Again, he was aware that this was taking things to the extreme, yet he could not stop himself.

We had a long, long talk that lasted well into the night. There was no doubt about his intelligence, but he did admit that since his wife had left him he had become obsessed with trivialities — anything to fill the emptiness of a lonely life. I really felt for him, as now that he had taken down his mask completely, he appeared more pathetic than eccentric.

With the help of a local doctor who was a very good friend of mine, we found him reliable accommodation with people who showed great understanding towards him. He seemed to be quite content there, being pampered and having all their attention lavished on him.

After he had stayed with these people for a few months or so, we received a note informing us that he had been offered a job in a maternity clinic and had decided to accept it. Our immediate reaction was: "Heaven help the mothers and babies there!"

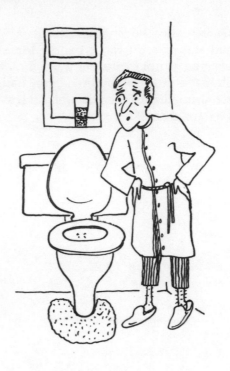

7

Red Alert

SLIGHTLY LESS traumatic than the incident concerning
Dr X was another call-out, also at night. It was during a
period when we were extremely busy and every available
bed in the clinic was occupied. We were working all hands
to the deck and it had been a long, long day, so I was happy
to finally go home and put my feet up.

I was already sound asleep when, well after midnight, a
new duty sister phoned to inform me that a certain new
patient had been greatly alarmed to find large amounts of
blood in his stools. She was extremely worried because he

seemed panic-stricken and urged me to attend the clinic immediately.

On arrival at the clinic, the sister explained that she had not been able to check the patient's story as he had, in his panic, flushed the evidence down the toilet. He had, however, been greatly agitated, as such a thing had never happened to him before.

When I spoke to the gentleman concerned and checked his records, I soon realised what had occurred. He had been admitted the previous day and it is customary that side-salads are served at lunch-time, always containing some beetroot. Moreover, it had been the first time this gentleman had tasted beetroot juice and he had liked it so much that he had requested an extra helping. In the mid-evening he had asked for yet another glass of beetroot juice. The explanation for the discoloration of his bowel movements was therefore simple!

It was an elementary matter of deduction that, unfortunately, cost me a few hours of precious sleep. However, the sooner a patient is reassured, the better. And I suppose that I would ten times rather have my sleep disturbed for such an unfortunate misunderstanding than for a serious emergency.

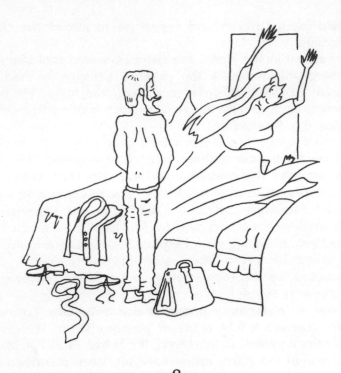

8

Unorthodox Methods

IN MY STUDENT days I developed quite an appreciative relationship with one of my tutors, a medical professor. He had been of great support to me during my training and I felt privileged that he continued to take an interest in my career. Because of this special bond between us, it was to him that I turned when I was confronted with a problem that I could not solve.

On this occasion, a new patient had been admitted to our clinic a few weeks previously. She was an extremely attractive young woman in her early twenties who had been bedridden for the last six months. Her parents had spent a small fortune on doctors' and specialists' fees, which fortunately they could well afford. Nevertheless, all the medical advice and reassurances they had received had not changed the situation one little bit. Tests had confirmed that everything was in order; their daughter's reflexes worked normally and yet it was cemented in her mind that she was unable to walk.

Therefore, in desperation, I turned to my favourite professor for advice. He listened patiently to my summary of her case history and asked a few pertinent questions. He then sat back and curled his moustache and stroked his beard, as he was wont to do when pondering on something. Eventually, he slowly rose from his chair, looked at me thoughtfully, and asked me to accompany him to the young lady's room. He stressed, however, that he wanted me to stay in the background. Under no circumstances was I to leave the room, as for propriety's sake it was essential that I remained present.

We made our way up the stairs and knocked on her door and she invited us to enter. She was half-sitting up in bed, looking as pretty as a picture. The professor made his way over to her and sat himself down on the edge of the bed. After I had introduced them to each other I moved back and stood behind a screen to watch.

They presented an interesting picture. There the professor sat, with his beautiful mop of silver hair and well-kept beard, looking very distinguished. The young lady was sitting up in bed, looking animated and a picture of health. She had brightened up remarkably as a result of the interest being focused on her. The professor remained on the edge of the bed talking to her, all the time gently stroking her hand, which she had innocently placed in his.

The conversation between them was pretty general and to be honest I was not paying full attention to what they were saying. I have to admit that I was slightly puzzled as to what he was trying to achieve. My ears pricked up somewhat when I heard him ask her if she was content to just lie there. Of course she denied this adamantly and a watchful expression crossed her face. The professor continued talking to her gently and I discovered a new slant to the conversation. He was telling her how young and lovely she looked and how she seemed so comfortable resting there. He, on the other hand, was growing old and weary — and wouldn't it be nice if they could share some experiences . . .

Talking all the while, he got up from the bed and took off his jacket, followed by his tie. Then he started undoing his shirt buttons. Looking at the girl, I saw her eyes open wider and wider as she watched him taking off his shirt. Then he proceeded to remove his shoes and finally started to unbutton his trousers, still talking non-stop.

I seem to recollect that he was by now in the process of explaining to her that his blood was getting thinner, the older he got, and that if he joined her in bed, she would keep him warm. The next thing I knew, there was a flurry of bedclothes and the young lady was up on her feet and running towards the door. This she wrenched open, screaming at the top of her voice.

Well, what can I say? The treatment method was certainly unorthodox. But then again, it worked!

It then became clear why the professor had been so insistent that I accompany him to the room and remain there, because it would indeed have been risky for him if his intentions had been misinterpreted or, rather, backfired, had I not been there as a witness.

Thank goodness, it had all worked out as planned. The girl realised that she had reacted in a perfectly normal manner and that her legs had not given way from under her. From that point she remained on her feet and her wasting muscles soon became stronger. Many a time since we have had a good laugh about the ingenuity of the wise old professor.

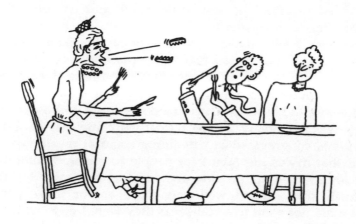

9

Conversation Stopper

DURING MY EARLY years of practising in Britain, we established a residential clinic on the west coast of Scotland. There was also a day clinic there and this part of the practice thrived to such an extent that in the end I had to choose between the clinic for out-patients and the residential clinic.

With the latter we were highly dependent on our staff, to such an extent that the unexpected absence of just one member of staff could throw a spanner in the works and affect the smooth running of the daily routine. In addition, the growing world-wide interest in alternative medicine was leading to ever more frequent invitations for me to give lectures abroad and attend international conferences and seminars. For these reasons I seemed to be spending more and more time away from home and therefore I finally decided to close the residential clinic and concentrate on attending to out-patients.

Indeed, I felt sorry at having to make this choice as, over the years, I had treated many patients under our roof, and their gratitude had often been heart-warming. Needless to say, I am still in touch with quite a few of our earlier patients and I have some very fond memories of those days.

It was customary in our residential clinic that all mobile patients congregated in the dining room at mealtimes. We felt that it was important for people to mix and communal meals seemed to provide the ideal opportunity for this. Mostly this worked well enough, even for those people who did not want to socialise, as they were free to withdraw to their own room between mealtimes and their therapy sessions. Many, however, made some very good friends during their stay with us.

I remember one old lady who had been admitted to the clinic for a therapy course that was meant to last for three weeks. I rather liked her, in fact, but had to admit that she did not blend in very well with the other patients who were at the clinic during her stay with us. The old lady was aware of this and therefore we offered her the option of having her meals served in her room. This she turned down as she was determined to stick it out.

Normally, some lively conversations and discussions were struck up at mealtimes and for the patients from abroad this proved an ideal opportunity to overcome any possible language barrier and integrate. Our little old lady, however, felt out of place and in her attempts to cover this up she became more gauche and even slightly abrasive or offensive. She clearly felt out of her depth, but refused to take the option of an easy way out.

At this point a high-ranking government official arrived to stay with us for a relatively short spell. On his first day it immediately became clear that he was an excellent conversationalist; he involved everyone round the table in the general discussion and solicited even the opinions of those who tended to be more timid.

However, our little old lady did not participate and, as I have said, tended to become rather curt through embarrassment. One mealtime, I happened to be moving about in the next room and caught snippets of the conversation while passing in and out of the dining room, when suddenly I was alerted by a series of screams.

I rushed back into the dining room where I noticed a great variety of facial expressions among the patients surrounding the old lady. Her own face was absolutely aghast. Her eyes looked as if they were about to pop out of their sockets and she had covered her mouth with both hands. Her fixed stare was focused on the dish of vegetables which had been placed in the middle of the table. Indeed, there in the dish, ensconced by the carrots, I could see her top set of dentures.

After the initial screams had subsided, and the silence that followed, pandemonium broke out. Everyone had some opinion on the unfortunate accident and did not hesitate to voice it. One member of staff smartly removed the vegetable dish with the offending contents and escorted the old lady from the dining room, while the rest of the staff apologised all round and attempted to regain some semblance of normality.

The old lady, however, was at the end of her tether. I learned that she had swallowed in embarrassment when the newcomer had addressed himself to her and choked on a piece of food. The strength of the cough which resulted had forced her dentures from her mouth. Unable to accept our reassurances that it could have happened to anyone, she insisted on phoning her son, who had brought her to the clinic, and then went to her room to pack her case. She left the clinic while the other patients were having supper, so that she did not have to face or speak to anyone again who had witnessed this unfortunate event.

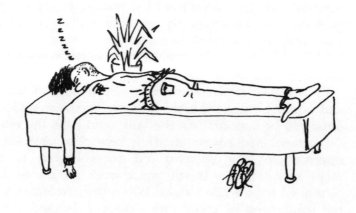

10

Ultimate Relaxation

ON ONE PARTICULARLY busy morning a gentleman in his early forties was shown into my consulting-room. He wore a tense and worried look on his face and appeared to be highly strung. He admitted that he had experienced trouble sleeping since his wife had left him for another man after having had a brief affair. I felt very sorry for him and would have liked to spend more time with him, but I had a waiting-room full of patients to attend to. I therefore asked him if he was in any hurry, because if he was not I could give up my lunch-break and spend some extra time with him. He was delighted with this suggestion and told me that he would "hang around" for the next hour or so.

Rather than see him bored, I put it to him that as he was so tense he might benefit from some relaxation. I checked and found that there were no other appointments for the remainder of the morning for the relaxation department. So at about half past eleven the gentleman disappeared up the stairs and I instructed the assistant as to what I had in mind for him. She could play one or two special relaxation tapes and also I suggested a neck massage.

By half past twelve there was still no sign of his return, and when I enquired after him my assistant said that he must still be upstairs. As the lady who runs the relaxation department had always made it very clear that she hated interruptions, my assistant did not volunteer to go and make sure. There was still more work for me to do, so I continued for a while longer. When the gentleman had still not reappeared by about one o'clock, I decided to risk the wrath of the relaxation department's assistant and go and see for myself.

I quietly knocked on the door and opened it just enough to poke my head round. The weirdest thoughts went through my mind when I peeped inside. The gentleman was lying on the treatment couch having his neck massaged. It would have presented a peaceful picture, if it had not been for the fact that his head seemed to be detached from his body. The assistant became aware of my presence and gently indicated that I should stay quiet. It was not until I had approached the couch and could hear the gentle snoring that I realised what was happening.

I have so far forgotten to mention that the lady in question had rather poor eyesight. This was no problem, as it did not affect her ability to do her work. In this instance, however, she was massaging the gentleman's neck, totally oblivious to the fact that he was wearing a wig — which had become dislodged. He, on the other hand, was sound asleep and at each of the assistant's strokes his wig popped up and then fell back again. In the sparse light of the treatment room, it had looked to me as if his head had become detached from the body; that is what had given me such a shock as I popped my head around the door.

The gentleman woke up when the regularity of the massage strokes ceased and when it was explained to him what had happened, he could see the funny side of it. He tidied himself up and then joined me in the library where indeed we had a good chat. He unburdened his problems and we decided on suitable tactics and a programme to help him further to overcome his anxiety. As an aside, he mentioned that he had just enjoyed the best sleep he had experienced for a long time!

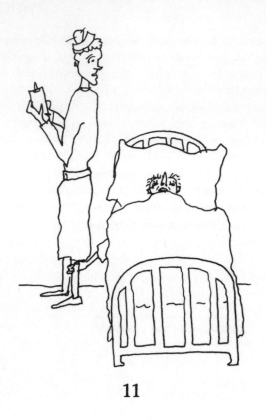

11

A Misfit

VERY OCCASIONALLY IT has happened that for some
reason or another we have had to ask a patient to leave
the residential clinic. A Dutch gentleman fell into this category. He was in his mid-forties and had decided to spend
his holiday in Scotland and have some medical conditions
attended to at the same time. He felt very pleased with
himself for being able to combine the two and arrived in an
exuberant mood at the clinic.

It did not take us long before we appreciated that we
might have a problem here. This gentleman's general atti-

tude left a great deal to be desired. At mealtimes he adopted a slightly superior attitude towards his fellow patients, while his approach to the staff was that of excessive familiarity. Amongst ourselves we discussed this character and we warily decided to keep a close eye on things, hoping that he would not upset any of the other patients.

Then one night, at three o'clock in the morning, I was woken by a telephone call from the clinic. The staff nurse asked me to come as she was having some unusual problems with our Dutch patient. He had called her several times during the late evening and night and had generally made a nuisance of himself. He had been making suggestive overtures and was not to be put off. When answering his latest call he had tried to force her into bed with him and she had now reached the point of refusing to answer any more of his calls. As the other staff on the night shift were all female, she had decided to call me, so that I could put this patient in his place.

I spoke sharply to the gentleman concerned and pointed out to him that if he wished to stay, he had to comply with the house rules and adopt a different attitude. He was fairly taken aback and expressed his surprise that his amorous attempts had been reported, but promised that it would not happen again.

Granted, no further nocturnal disturbances were reported and we tried to settle down to a pattern. However, he blotted his copybook yet again. Because of a specific health problem he had been fitted with a portable urinal and one lunch-time he produced this in the dining room and made it generally understood that he was prepared to relieve himself there and then. He was quickly escorted out of the room and the incident was reported to me.

This was the straw that broke the camel's back. He was told that we were not able to cater for him any longer at our establishment, owing to his anti-social behaviour. If he chose to do so, he was still allowed to attend the clinic for his therapy sessions, but would have to stay at one of the local hotels. We offered to phone around to obtain accommodation for him, but he definitely could not stay with us any longer because of his disruptive behaviour.

I must admit that when he decided to discharge himself, no one expressed any grief at his departure.

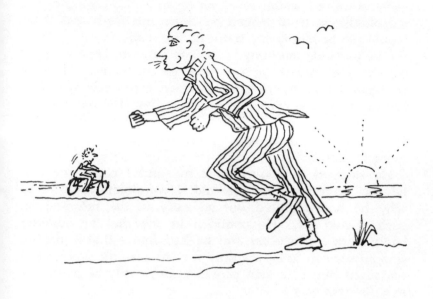

12

The Early Bird

AS FAR BACK as I can remember, I have always been in the habit of rising early in the morning. It still stands me in good stead. Most mornings I am at my desk well before seven o'clock and I use this time to attend to administrative matters. It is a time when one is rarely interrupted and therefore much can be achieved in a relatively short period. Once the first patient arrives we are usually kept busy until well into the evening.

During the days that the clinic was still a residential establishment, I would arrive there on my bicycle at around six o'clock in the morning. The short trip from my home to the clinic would take me along the golf course and each morning I would revel yet again at the beauty of my surroundings. It all looked so clean and fresh and there would still be hardly any traffic on the roads.

One particular morning in the late autumn, I saw a jogger on the golf course on my way to the clinic. I quickly recognised him as being the German gentleman who had booked in at the clinic the previous day. He was jogging along in his pyjama jacket, with an anxious look on his face. I called out to him in his own language: "Guten morgen, Herr S!"

He stopped to acknowledge me and I could see that he was shivering from the cold. I wondered aloud as to why he had ventured out so early in the morning on such a cold day. He confided in me that he suffered badly from constipation and he had found that a jogging session seemed to be the only way to ease his problems. I reassured him that such problems can easily be overcome in a different way.

We met again after breakfast and he told me that his problems had become more pronounced after some drastic set-backs in his career and further difficulties in his private life. I had previously heard the expression "having a constipated look about him", but would find it difficult to define. This gentleman, however, as I remember him, fitted the description exactly.

As promised, we easily solved his problems with the help of a natural remedy and an adjustment to his diet. Thereafter, he considered himself fortunate at not having to go jogging early each morning, irrespective of the weather.

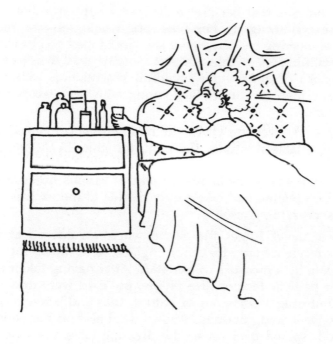

13

A Doctor's Nightmare

ONE MORNING AT around breakfast-time I received a telephone call from a local general practitioner. He asked me how I was placed for time that day, as he would appreciate it if I could accompany him to see a patient of his. With his knowledge and co-operation, I had already been consulted previously by this patient, and therefore he wanted me to be involved.

The patient in question was a well-to-do middle-aged lady, who was terribly unhappy. Not having a definite goal in life, she suffered largely imaginary problems in an effort to gain attention. She had become a dedicated hypochondriac and had several strings to her bow. She would see one doctor and, on hearing his diagnosis, she would then go elsewhere for confirmation of that judgement. She was therefore on the books of quite a few medical practitioners, although basically there was not a lot wrong with her, except utter boredom.

However, over the years she had become convinced that the more tablets or pills she took, the more likely she was to be cured. Her life now revolved round the clock, as she had so many medicines to take at various times of the day. This regime had taken over her life to the exclusion of almost everything else.

I will never forget the scene when we arrived at this lady's residence later that morning and were shown into her bedroom by a member of her staff. After having taken note of her pathetic face on the pillow, my eyes were drawn to the confusing assortment of bottles, tubs and boxes of pills and tablets, and goodness knows what else on her bedside table. It spilled over on to the dressing table and even on to the floor. The table surfaces were literally stacked with remedies, supposedly meant to help her regain her physical and mental health. She seemed to be a total wreck and looked pathetically helpless.

Her doctor and I sat down and prepared ourselves for a long talk with her. We pointed out that she was ruining her health with this obsessive pill-popping and I expressed surprise that she had not "exploded" as a result of inter-reactions between the great variety of chemicals she was ingesting in the multitude of pills and tablets she regularly took. This expression seemed to tickle her sense of humour, because she repeated it several times.

Luckily, it was not yet too late to help this lady. She listened to our warnings and accepted our advice and came to the conclusion that she had to take herself in hand. Both her doctor and myself kept a close eye on her and slowly she was weaned off the addictive habits she had developed and that had been threatening to destroy her.

I still see this particular lady every now and then and she always makes a point of laughingly reassuring me that there is no chemical warfare going on in her body, so an "explosion" is most unlikely!

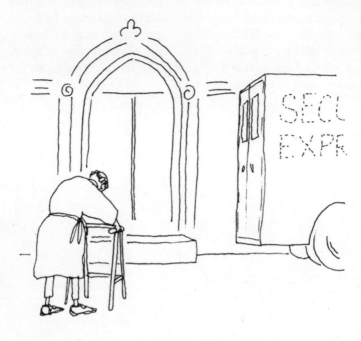

14

Taken for a Ride

CONTRARY TO POPULAR belief, the life of an alternative practitioner is not exactly rosy. It is true that the gratitude of patients is extremely rewarding, but on the other hand we also suffer from the stigma of being referred to as "cranks" at best, and "opportunists" at worst. Especially in the earlier days, many patients who would call on our expertise, would do so only as a last resort. They would do the rounds of the orthodox medical establishments and would then end up on our doorsteps with the attitude: "Nothing ventured, nothing gained!"

More recently I have become aware of a slightly more liberal attitude, but certainly in those early days the financial situation was often fraught within our establishment and we continually had to prove our worth. The process of having to persuade people to believe that "liquidised grass" — as I have heard people refer to homoeopathic herbal preparations — has remedial benefits, has at times been arduous to say the least.

Alternative medicine is extremely diverse. Not only are herbal drops and tablets used, but dietary adaptations are advised and many therapies that were, and still are, considered unorthodox have proved to be successful. Take acupuncture, for example; over the last few years this has more or less become a household word.

However, going back to those early days, it was not uncommon for me to treat an occasional "doubting Thomas" free of charge. When I know instinctively that I can alleviate the suffering of a patient, I have never been able to turn him away and leave him to get on with it. If I recognised a willingness to be helped, but realised that it would be a struggle for that individual to pay for the required remedies, I have sometimes lowered the price or given the treatment free of charge.

One of my "Good Samaritan" exercises, however, left me with egg on my face and this experience is definitely listed in my book as a lesson for the future.

One sunny afternoon I saw a blue van pull up in the car park. The rear door was opened and an elderly gentleman was helped into a wheelchair and wheeled into the reception area of the clinic by a young driver. The wheelchair was left there by the young man, who returned to the van to wait.

I thought it strange that the elderly gentleman made no effort to confirm his arrival with the receptionist and approached him to ask what time his appointment was. He replied that he had not made an appointment but that he was severely crippled by rheumatism and near enough incapable of movement. His general practitioner had tried everything possible but he had reached the end of the road. He now wondered if there was anything that I could do for him. However, he hastened to add that as his pension did not leave him with a penny to spare, would I consider using him as a guinea-pig to see if alternative methods could help where orthodox medicine had been found lacking.

I told him that we were by no means miracle workers and that the treatment he appeared to need would be rather expensive. However, he reiterated that there was no way at all that he could pay me for my trouble. I looked at the poor fellow and decided that I would help him, although I could not see him that particular afternoon. We made an appointment for him, called back his driver, and off he went.

A fortnight later he arrived for his appointment and we checked his overall physical condition and gathered notes for his case history. He suffered from other complaints besides rheumatoid arthritis and the regular treatment he required would take most of an afternoon. Not only was the treatment lengthy, it was also labour-intensive. A physiotherapist would be heavily involved, as would a nurse. He also needed mud baths, acupuncture treatment, manipulation and several remedies.

For a long period he attended the clinic twice a week — free of charge. I admit that he co-operated well with his diet and did his utmost to be punctual. He really made such incredible progress that he became mobile again, albeit that he needed a stick for walking. When we had reached this stage, I asked him if it was at all possible for him to reimburse me for some of the medication, as there had been a considerable price increase due to a fluctuation in the foreign exchange rates.

He took offence at this and pointed out that he had already told me that this was impossible. Finally, I reassured him that the treatment would be continued, but as he had made such fantastic progress, I suggested that a fortnightly treatment session would be sufficient if he continued to take care. He was adamant that this would not be enough and by this time I was beginning to lose my patience somewhat and reminded him that there were many other people in equal need of treatment, if not more.

He did not appear for his next appointment and actually we were sorry that he did not turn up for his regular treatment as he had been progressing so well. There was no doubt in our minds that he would have soon been able to walk again without the aid of his stick.

About five months later I met him at the local bus station and was pleasantly surprised at how well he could move about. When I asked him why he had not returned to the clinic he told me that he was scared that I would insist on payment. I assured him that after all that time it was hardly likely I was going to do such a thing. We were actually all very proud of him because he had made such fantastic progress.

Twelve months later he turned up again at the clinic, shuffling about with the aid of two sticks — it could hardly be called walking. He was very apologetic, but felt that he had to let me know that he had not even been able to afford the diet that I had recommended for him. I pointed out that he must have realised how important that dietary regime was for his condition and agreed to take him back for treatment. However, he did not appear at his appointed time and I did not see him again.

Quite some time after that I arrived home one evening, absolutely worn out. I had a quick glance through the paper before retiring to bed. A caption caught my eye about somebody who had left the grand sum of £2,750,000 in his will. It concerned an elderly person with a fairly common name, but some alarm bells started ringing in my mind. I told my wife that I had just the faintest suspicion that this was the gentleman who had arrived in the blue van, although that did not add up with what I knew of him. My curiosity was aroused by now and, forgetting my fatigue, I went back to the clinic to check his address in the files.

To my utter surprise and, I must admit it, also my abhorrence, I realised that, indeed, this was the very same man.

This was the gentleman who had pleaded poverty so frequently and who, despite his progress, had chosen to discontinue the treatment for fear of being asked to pay towards its cost.

It struck me that an apt epitaph on his tombstone might have been: "Here lies the man who loved his money more than his health." Though, come to think of it, he would have hated the thought of spending money on a tombstone in the first place!

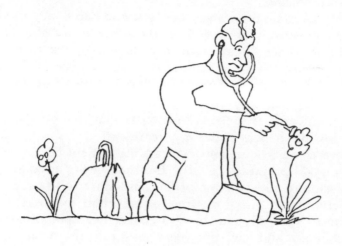

15

Prejudice

I HAVE ALREADY made reference to the fact that practising alternative medicine is not always an enviable occupation. We practitioners often have to live with an attitude of condescending superiority on the part of our orthodox counterparts. Mostly this is based on a lack of knowledge concerning our specialised field and sometimes on misunderstanding but, worst of all, it can be due to a "closed mind".

When I am faced with professional disbelief and lack of co-operation, I often think back to one particular incident, with a certain measure of glee. The patient concerned was a middle-aged woman who was married to a successful hospital specialist. She had come to me after having exhausted all the orthodox medical avenues without finding a solution to her problems.

With a certain reluctance, her husband had finally yielded to her pressure and agreed to allow her to try alternative medicine. After I had made my diagnosis, the treatment soon proved to be effective and she co-operated well. Nevertheless, she informed me that her husband, though recognising her improvement and sharing in her delight, still considered it to be coincidental that this should take place while she was under my treatment.

Several visits were needed, but the patient continued to make good progress. Usually, the time of her appointment was set from mid- to late-morning, in order to give her ample opportunity to arrive in time, as she had to travel a fair distance. One day she had to cancel her appointment at short notice and she later filled me in on the details as to why she had not been able to keep it.

On that particular trip she had been joined by her husband and a colleague of his together with his wife. It had been decided to make a day of it. After she had attended the clinic for her appointment, they intended to tour the countryside and stop somewhere for lunch. Unfortunately, before they managed to reach the clinic they ran into unforeseen problems. The car they were travelling in stalled and refused to go any further. Beautiful countryside it may have been, but it was also very sparsely populated and they needed help. They eventually noticed a farm in the distance and there seemed no alternative but to lock up the car and walk to the farm and ask to be allowed to use the phone to get some help.

When they arrived at the farm they ran into further problems. The farmer proved totally unco-operative and refused them entry, as he had too often been taken for granted by people who had arrived on his doorstep with tales of woe. He curtly told them to leave his premises. My patient's husband then asked that even if he did not allow them to contact a garage or motoring organisation to get help for their stranded vehicle, would he please let them make a telephone call to Troon, as his wife had a doctor's appointment there and he would be happy to reimburse the farmer for the cost of the call.

My patient then told me that both doctors had expressed great surprise at the farmer's reaction. The farmer had hesitantly enquired: "Do you mean the Dutch doctor in Troon?" They confirmed this and at that the farmer changed his tune. He invited them into the house, told them where the phone was and asked his wife to put on the kettle.

As they waited for a mechanic to come and see to the car, over a cup of tea the farmer told them about the miracles this Dutch doctor had performed for him and asked would they kindly remember him to the doctor and once again express his gratitude. He stressed that if it had not been for that Dutch doctor he would not have been able to continue farming.

The two gentlemen in particular listened attentively to the recollections of the farmer concerning his treatment at our clinic and then they informed him of their profession. The farmer bluntly gave them his opinion of orthodox medicine. He told how he had been sent from pillar to post and all to no avail. No, to his way of thinking, the Dutch doctor knew what it was all about!

All this was related to me by the doctor's wife and she added that they had not even been allowed to pay for the telephone calls. On a subsequent visit she told me happily that the other good thing that had transpired from this unplanned diversion, was that her husband had stopped criticising alternative medicine.

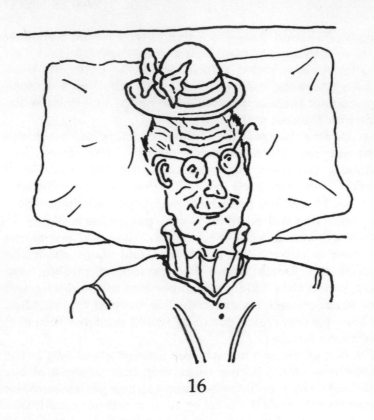

16

Short Treatment

ALTHOUGH I DO not often accept lunch-time engage-
ments, on this occasion I had made an exception. By
popular request I had been invited to give a talk at a Rotary
Club luncheon and immediately afterwards I returned to the
clinic to start a very busy afternoon surgery.

My first patient that afternoon was a dear old lady who
had been a patient of ours for a long time. She was a
farmer's wife who suffered very badly from osteo-arthritis,
particularly in her knees. When she felt really in need, she
would phone to make an appointment for acupuncture

treatment and that way we managed to keep her going. She was a very gentle and pleasant person and never very demanding, which especially endeared her to the staff. Always very punctual for her appointment, she also showed great appreciation for the relief of her pain after the visits.

This afternoon, as always, she was wearing her little bonnet which she never took off for her acupuncture treatment. I remarked that she was looking rather pale and wan that day and she told me that she had been very busy and had also been off her food. We chatted away while I positioned the acupuncture needles and I decided to check her blood pressure. Nothing out of the ordinary was found, nor with her heartbeat. I then left my principal physiotherapist in charge, but shortly afterwards was called back, as she was not happy with the patient's condition.

I immediately realised that our patient was about to faint and although we took preventive action, she went out like a light. When I took her pulse again it was only very slight and my physiotherapist could not locate anything stronger. We were baffled and becoming increasingly concerned. We had just reached the decision that an ambulance should be called, when she opened her eyes.

Now, imagine this dear little face with the bonnet still planted on her head, albeit slightly askew, as were her spectacles: there was not much of her, but she looked even frailer lying there, with the colour drained from her face.

When she had opened her eyes, she asked in her kind and gentle voice: "Is that it for today? It seems to have gone so quickly."

She actually sounded rather disappointed and clearly had no idea how much anxiety she had caused and was totally unaware that she had passed out during her treatment. Not noticing the beads of perspiration on our faces, caused by our frantic efforts to revive her, she remarked with a friendly smile that it had been a very good treatment today and that she felt very relaxed.

We helped her up and explained to her what had happened. She then apologised for all the trouble she had inadvertently caused and we took her to an ante-room where she could have a quiet cup of tea. After having heard what had happened, she was ready to accept our advice that she must take things a little easier and take better care of herself. Some of the work would just have to be left until another time and she had to slow down a bit. Don't we all, when growing older, have to accept the fact that we are not spring chickens anymore and therefore do not quite have the physical stamina of an eighteen-year-old?

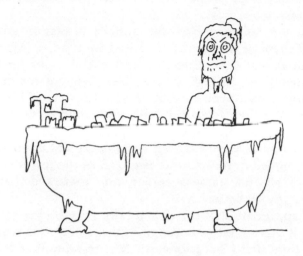

17

A Cold Spell

IN THE EARLIER days of building up my practice in Scotland, it happened occasionally that I would visit a patient in his or her home if that was especially requested. Yet even in those days it was an exception to the rule and during more recent years home visits have been totally out of the question, as the surgery is fully booked well in advance.

Before the clinic became so busy, however, I remember one occasion when I received a telephone call asking me to visit an elderly female patient at home. Her family told me that she had spent a badly disturbed night and that their doctor had merely told them that the problem would very likely sort itself out, but to keep him informed nonetheless. When I saw the patient she was in great distress and had a dangerously high temperature, which was causing her to be delirious.

I could not fail to notice the family's hesitation when I informed them of the treatment I had in mind. I reassured them that it would be effective and asked them for their full co-operation. At my request they brought me half-a-dozen large bath towels and all the ice they could lay their hands on. We then filled the bath with ice-cold water and lifted the patient into the bath and placed ice packs around her body. As we were bathing her the patient opened her eyes and looked at us without any sign of the feverous hallucinations she had shown earlier, and remarked that she now felt so much better.

I fully appreciate that this is a totally unorthodox therapy and that it takes a bit of courage to use it, but this was not the first time that I had done so. My grandmother always maintained that this was the most effective way to break a fever; bathing the body with cold water will always reduce a temperature and in this case the temperature had been raging so high that drastic action had been required.

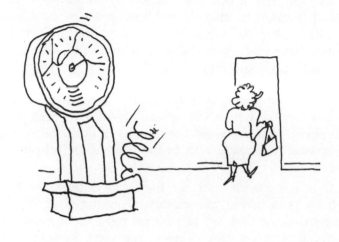

18

A Weighty Problem

SO OFTEN IT surprises me that people are loath to accept
any responsibility for their own health. It is the most
precious thing we will ever have — the gift of life. Why
then do we not take better care of it? It is infinitely easier
to maintain good health, than to regain it once lost, and often
all that is required is a matter of good common sense.

A new patient was shown into my consulting-room and
I perceived what I estimated to be a lady of middle age,
of very ample proportions and with an extremely florid
complexion. There she sat, opposite me, gasping for breath.

When I asked her the reason for her visit, she told me that her doctor had been most insistent that she lose weight, for her own good. However, so far she had found it impossible.

Even as she sat there she became yet redder in the face and I was not sure if this was caused by embarrassment or anxiety. I decided to check her blood pressure and while doing this I asked her what age she was. She told me that she was thirty-eight years old and at the same time I read on the sphygmomanometer that her blood pressure was 210 / 150. Her heart was beating away like a hammer — as I imagine any practitioner might have done if they had a patient like her in the consulting-room, I sent up an urgent prayer that she would remain alive until she had left the premises. She really was in the most dreadful physical condition.

As it is not uncommon for high blood pressure to be caused by poor bowel movements, I enquired about this. She informed me that her last bowel movement must have been about a week ago. Maybe we were getting somewhere . . .

We reviewed her dietary management and I gave her some suggestions for a more healthy way of eating. This would be beneficial not only from the point of view of losing weight, but also in that she would receive sufficient fibre. I explained to her the importance of this substance for ensuring regular bowel movements and, finally, prescribed some natural remedies and explained the benefits of administering an enema and instructed her accordingly.

She returned a fortnight later, proudly telling me about her weight loss. She looked much better in the face already and her blood pressure had also improved greatly. She also remarked that her headaches had almost disappeared and wanted to know if that could also be ascribed to the laxatives. I agreed that this was likely to be the case and pointed out to her that the constipation and obesity had placed unnecessary strain on her heart and caused high blood pressure, which in turn would have triggered the headaches. If she was sensible her problems would soon be a thing of the past and she would be able to look back with a sense of satisfaction and achievement.

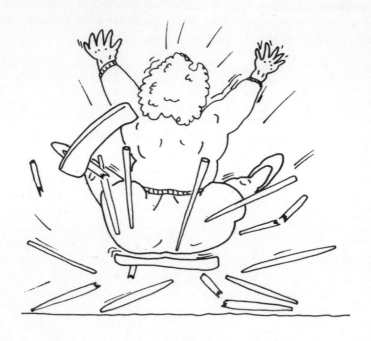

19

All Blunders

COMING BACK TO common sense, I must point out that a great lack of this can often be observed among those patients who seek our help in order to lose weight. A perfect example of this was one particular extremely overweight patient who weighed in excess of twenty stones.

On her first visit she planted herself on to a chair that promptly collapsed underneath her. When she had been helped to her feet she had the audacity to say, with an indignant look on her face, that the chair must have been "wonky" as it could not hold her. Politely, I pointed out to her that it could possibly have been her weight, refraining from stressing the point that she had not actually sat down in a normal manner, but had let herself fall down on to the chair as her freedom of movement was greatly hampered by her obesity.

When she was asked to step on to the scales and told what her weight amounted to, she stated, with a perfectly straight face, that the scales must be out of order as her weight was well below the figure we mentioned. Nevertheless, we discussed a dietary regime with her and arranged a second appointment for a fortnight later.

When she returned two weeks later she was weighed again. On being told that she had not lost one single ounce, she calmly stated that she had warned us that she was a special case — and obviously the diet we had suggested was not suitable for her. In an effort to help her adhere to the diet, we then prescribed a herbal remedy and instructed her on its use.

Another fortnight later she came back for her next appointment. Again, when she was weighed it was discovered that she had not lost any weight whatsoever. This time her immediate sullen answer was that the pills she had been prescribed were obviously no good at all.

It was very clear to us that this patient had adopted the mental attitude that everything and everyone was to blame for her obesity except herself.

After that third visit we put our heads together and decided to give her one last chance, but if she turned up for her next appointment still not having lost any weight, we would have to inform her that we were not able to help her unless she was prepared to help herself. We were saved the trouble because she never appeared for her appointment and we never saw her again.

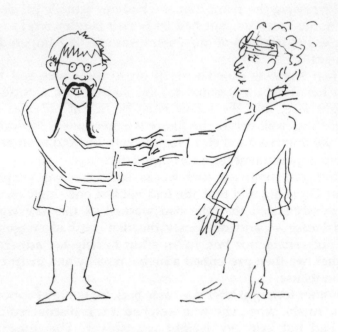

20

East–West Trade

MY ACUPUNCTURE STUDIES took place in China and I was very surprised to encounter a great amount of secrecy among the practitioners there. I found this to be particularly so among successful acupuncturists, who tended to guard the exact position of their individual acupuncture points with a tremendous professional secrecy. Conditions are different in China and it is often a hard struggle for newly qualified individuals to establish a practice.

Acupuncture can be used for a tremendous variety of purposes. To name but a few, it can serve as an anaesthetic during surgical operations, or as a means of pain relief, and recently it has been used very successfully to help people overcome addictive habits. When I say recently, I would like you to realise that acupuncture has been practised in China for many, many centuries. However, addictions to alcohol, nicotine or other drugs can now be dealt with effectively by acupuncture treatment.

During my time in China, I noticed that one particular Chinese doctor organised anti-smoking sessions several times daily and each time the sessions were fully booked. Word of his successful treatment methods had spread widely and more and more people queued to be included in these therapy sessions.

The little Chinese doctor just went about his business as usual with a permanent enigmatic smile on his face. Despite being so popular, he had no assistant to relieve him of some of his workload — and I soon realised the reason for this. During several conversations with him it became quite clear to me that he was not going to divulge the exact locations of the points where he placed the needles. That was his very own trade secret and that was the way he preferred it to remain.

Herbal remedies have always been very popular in China and we often talked on the subject. I have already mentioned that I come from a long line of naturopathic practitioners and, moreover, I have been trained by one of the greatest, namely Dr Alfred Vogel from Switzerland. It came about that one particular remedy was being discussed between us and before I quite realised what was happening, the Chinese doctor bent towards me secretly and, with his voice reduced to a whisper, asked me if it would be at all possible to grow the necessary herbs in China.

It was then that I realised that here was the opportunity for a bit of bartering. I suggested to him that I would not only send him the relevant herbs, but also instruct him on the formula used to prepare the specific remedy. However, I needed a favour in return. He looked at me dubiously when I indicated that I would like to be told which acupuncture points he used in his treatment to help smokers to overcome their addiction.

He hesitated for a moment, then grabbed my hand and started pumping it, indicating that we had a deal. I was subsequently invited to come to his consulting-rooms, where he would instruct me in the correct placement of the needles for that particular purpose.

My part of the deal was to share the successful formula with him, which I duly did. On my return to Europe I sent him the promised herbs and we still remain in touch with each other to this day

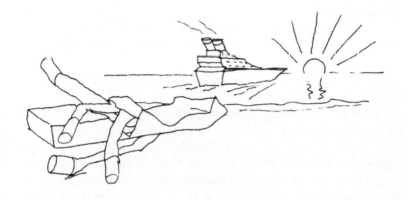

21

The Pep Talk

THE INSIDE INFORMATION I had obtained with such cunning concerning the exact positions in which to place the acupuncture needles to encourage patients to stop smoking, has benefited countless numbers of patients in the United Kingdom. At any one treatment session I usually treat about half-a-dozen patients, who all lie comfortably stretched out on a couch in a large, pleasantly decorated room.

I move about between the patients and while positioning the needles I quietly tell them what they are supposed to do. I tell them to think positively and repeat quietly to themselves that they will never, never smoke again. I ask them to repeat this promise to themselves over and over again.

During one such session I heard a middle-aged gentleman audibly repeat this phrase over and over to himself: "I will never smoke again. I will never smoke again. I will never smoke again."

Gradually his voice became somewhat more penetrating: "Darn it, *I will not* smoke again! *I must not* smoke again!"

Then, with a higher pitch to his voice: "Why did I start this filthy habit? If I had never started, I would not now have to go through this."

His voice dropping again he continued to repeat: "I will not smoke again. I will never smoke again."

It was obvious that quite involuntarily he was trying to hypnotise himself into giving up the habit. He actually got himself so worked up that eventually I had to take him out of the room and ask him to lie on the couch in the adjacent room, where I went through the whole procedure again. After the treatment session he left with an inspired look on his face and vowed to me that he would *never* smoke again.

What a delight it was to receive a postcard from him some time later with the message on it that he had successfully managed to give up smoking and as a result he had now, for the first time in his life, managed to save enough money to take his wife on a world cruise — where they were having the time of their lives!

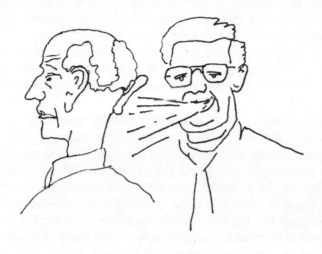

22

The Discarded Hearing-Aid

ANOTHER PROUD EXAMPLE of successful acupuncture treatment concerned a lovely old gentleman who was extremely hard of hearing. Initially he had come to me in desperation about his hearing ability, which seemed to be disappearing rapidly. He had cheered up considerably when I told him that we might be able to help him. I had to inform him, however, that it might take quite a few treatment sessions. Even though he had to travel a fair distance to keep his appointments, nothing would deter him if I thought that there was the slightest chance of any improvement.

Once the treatment had started a slight improvement was certainly noticeable, although it was still virtually impossible to have a conversation with him when his hearing-aid was switched off. Out of sheer enthusiasm, he would turn down the volume of the hearing-aid as if to prove that the treatment was being successful, but he would give the oddest answers to any questions I put to him.

I remember asking him once if he drank at all and he replied with an apologetic smile that that was not possible because of his hearing disability. I must have looked dumbfounded by this answer and my assistant actually started to giggle slightly, so he asked if I would repeat the question. When I did so, in a loud and clear manner, he smiled embarrassedly and explained that he had misunderstood me: he thought that I had asked him if he drove a car.

This might possibly sound an odd excuse for not driving, but I could well understand that he considered driving to be impossible because of his disability. I have had the same response from other people who were hard of hearing. It is something one rarely stops and thinks about if one has no hearing problems oneself, but with a hearing defect it is often very difficult to ascertain from which direction any sound is coming. Therefore one would be greatly confused when hearing a siren while driving along, not knowing from which direction the ambulance, fire engine or police car was approaching. This gentleman obviously considered himself a hazard to the traffic, as a result of his disability.

When he had been receiving treatment for some time, he took the chance one day of turning up for his appointment without his hearing-aid, as he was so proud of his improved hearing. He walked into the reception area and in a loud voice he announced his arrival. He then proceeded to enquire after the receptionist's health and volunteered that he himself was in excellent spirits. All this took place in an exaggeratedly loud voice. He went on to inform her that the doctor's treatment had been so effective that now he could manage without his hearing-aid. This last comment caused great hilarity among the other people in the waiting-room, as he could be heard all along the ground floor of the clinic.

To this gentleman, however, the long-forgotten experience of being able to hear the telephone ring or the doorbell, was reason enough for great excitement!

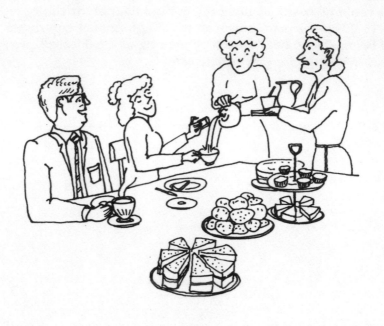

23

Do You Take Sugar?

NOT LONG AFTER I had opened my clinic in Scotland, a lady arrived from one of the islands that are dotted along the west coast of Scotland. The rugged beauty of these islands has to be seen to be fully appreciated, and over the years I have come to value their inhabitants greatly. They are straightforward, hospitable and loyal, and thanks to this female patient who stayed at our clinic in those early days, I have treated many, many more patients from the island since that time.

This particular lady arrived at the clinic by car and

was carried in, as she was unable to walk. She was a farmer's wife and for almost a year she had been an invalid. Extensive tests had been carried out, but no reason for her inability to walk could be pinpointed. A letter from her doctor stated that her illness was not psychosomatic and he feared that her condition was serious, although he did not know what exactly was wrong with her.

We installed her in a lovely room overlooking the sea and did our best to make her feel at home. Her family all lived on the island, so visiting was not easily arranged, but she was greatly loved by them and they did their utmost to come and see her whenever they could. She was a lovely patient to care for, because she was of a sunny disposition and so appreciative of everything that was done for her. She was therefore a great hit with the staff.

She stayed with us for quite some time and we started by conducting all the necessary tests, but her lower limbs appeared to be almost lifeless. We gave her massages and vibratory treatment, but it was thanks to acupuncture that we noticed the first faint reactions. Her treatment included herbal remedies and supplementary vitamins, minerals and trace elements and eventually things began to look up. She was certainly most co-operative and was very keen to follow every piece of advice she was given.

Some time during her treatment, she told me one day that her legs were beginning to feel as if they were part of her again. I promised her that very soon we would be going for a walk together and she laughed wistfully as if she could not quite believe that, no matter how much she would have liked to.

Sure enough, the day came that she managed the few steps necessary to cross the hallway, albeit heavily supported. That was the first major hurdle. She now realised that she would be able to walk again and was most anxious to improve on the progress already achieved.

Shortly afterwards, on a beautiful sunny spring morning, I opened the French doors of the treatment room and we stepped into the garden. Her sheer happiness and delight at her progress was touching to see.

This lady may have been carried off the island, but she did manage to return to it on her feet. Everyone was delighted, not least herself. She regularly returned to the clinic for follow-up treatment, but maintained a steady improvement.

During one of her short stays for further treatment, she brought along a friend of hers who was also ailing and between them they livened up the other patients. They were a treat to have with us, and I thoroughly enjoyed their stay.

Both ladies were involved in the island's branch of the SWRI (Scottish Women's Rural Institute) in an office-bearing capacity. Her recovery therefore did not go unnoticed and, to satisfy the islanders' curiosity, it was decided that I should give a talk to the ladies of the SWRI. As it turned out, the talk was attended by many people who had no connection with the SWRI and it was considered to have been a great success.

I have already mentioned that the islanders are very hospitable — and I should know, because I have been on the receiving end. It was typical that after the talk an impressive spread was laid on. The table groaned under the weight of home-cooking and baking. Ladies moved among the crowd offering coffee and tea and everyone was invited to help themselves to the food.

While I was sitting having a chat with the branch president, our cups were refilled and the tea lady was followed by a dear old lady carrying a tray with milk and sugar. She asked us if we took sugar and the president turned to her and said: "No thank you, dear, I have Hermesetas."

A shocked look came over the face of the little old lady and she replied: "Och dearie, I didnae ken that ye were nae well."

All this, of course, was greeted with great hilarity by some of the bystanders, who realised that she did not know that Hermesetas is not some dreaded disease, but merely an artificial sweetener!

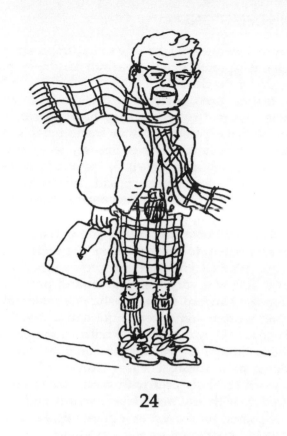

24

That Undeniable Accent

FOR ALMOST TWENTY years now I have lived and worked in Scotland and whenever this fact comes up in conversation, I am often asked why I came here in the first place. Well, that is easily answered: my wife is a Scot and although the earlier years of our marriage were spent in my native country, we eventually decided to move to Scotland. As much as I love my own country, the Netherlands, this is a decision that I have never regretted. I have a great affinity for Scotland and its people and that love has developed over the years into a feeling of belonging. I readily admit that it may not necessarily be one's first impression, but I have first-hand experience of the warmth, kindness, hospitality and loyalty of the Scots.

For that matter, I recognise these traits in Scots wherever I meet them. No matter where they have settled, most of them seem to have preserved that friendliness and sense of humour which I have come to appreciate so much over the years. I am often approached by expatriate Scots in the audience on my lecture tours abroad, especially when in Canada and the United States, and nearly always we seem to recognise a mutual appreciation.

I remember one occasion, quite some time ago now, when I was invited to take part in a public lecture in Los Angeles. When I checked the programme, I realised that I was to follow a very well-known and popular public speaker, namely Gaylord Hauser, who is a remarkable person and has written some very informative books, which are widely read. He was also an excellent example of what he preached, though by no means could he, even then, be considered as a spring chicken. Nevertheless, he continued to work tirelessly and with great vitality and would keep up to date with any new developments and whenever his name appeared on the list as a guest speaker at a public lecture, it would guarantee a good attendance.

When I learned that I was to follow Gaylord Hauser on the platform, I became rather worried. What would I do if people prepared to leave the assembly hall when he had finished his contribution? I need not have worried. Even though he was then in his eighties, he gave an inspired talk and judging from the reaction of the audience, as usual, it was greatly appreciated. He finished his allotted time by introducing me in the warmest of manners and, thank goodness, there was no mass exodus when he left the platform and took a seat at the front of the lecture hall. There he settled down to listen and although I had previously felt inadequate, this was of great encouragement to me.

I started my address by apologising in advance for my

accent and possibly slightly limited vocabulary. When I speak to a completely new audience for the first time I sometimes do this, and in this instance I certainly considered such an explanation necessary as I was to follow such an accomplished public speaker. My stage-fright quickly disappeared and as usual I warmed to my subject and settled down.

Afterwards, I was approached by an elderly gentleman who told me in a thick Scottish brogue that he originally hailed from Glasgow, although he had been living in California for well over twenty years. Appreciatively, he placed his hand on my shoulder and told me that hearing my Scottish accent had made his day.

Is it any wonder, then, that where I live I am sometimes referred to as MacVries?

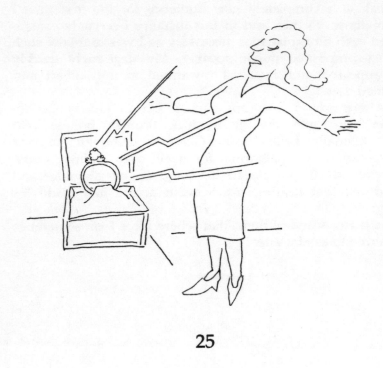

25

Telling Vibrations?

ON ANOTHER OCCASION, after I had spoken at a public meeting in a rural area, I was approached by a lady and gentleman. They had been sitting in the second row and I had noticed at the time that they had both been listening very attentively and with great concentration. They sought permission to ask me a personal question and of course I was prepared to listen to them. They wanted to know if I believed in energy vibrations.

Well, as acupuncture is a form of energy vibration and I have witnessed the results of this science in my practice over many years, I naturally told them that I most definitely did believe in energy vibrations, even though the subject is still shrouded by a lot of mysticism.

Once they realised I was sympathetic, the lady then proceeded to tell me that, over the last eighteen months or so, she had started to suffer from unusual and uncharacteristic epileptic fits. She had never been troubled with ill-health until after her mother had died. She had had a very strained relationship with her mother, but had experienced great happiness in her marriage. However, as a token of respect to her departed mother, she had decided to wear her mother's ring since her death.

From the onset of her ill-health she had sought medical attention, but the problems had arisen and increased in frequency. Only recently had she quite by chance discovered that when she was not wearing her mother's ring she generally felt better and was not subject to epileptic fits. She had discussed with her husband the possibility of there being any connection between her wearing her mother's ring and her sudden epileptic fits. Both of them were greatly puzzled by the whole phenomenon.

Without hesitation, I advised her to dispose of her mother's ring. She could sell it, or give it away — it didn't matter what she decided to do with it — but she should not wear it again. Some time afterwards she contacted me to let me know that since she had sold the ring, she had not encountered any further health problems.

This case is very similar to that of a gentleman in his mid-twenties who told me that he had inherited some money from a relative with whom he had never seen eye to eye. Most people would have considered themselves fortunate with such a nice little windfall, but ever since he had been informed of this inheritance, he had left the money untouched as he felt a certain aversion to spending it. He had grown anxious and troubled about this and asked me for my advice.

Just as I had told the lady to dispose of her mother's ring, here again my advice was ruthless. I advised him to give it to charity. Let people in the Third World benefit from it. That money could alleviate the suffering endured by less fortunate people while at the same time it would most likely make him a happier person in himself.

The young man took my advice and almost immediately he regained his usual cheerful nature.

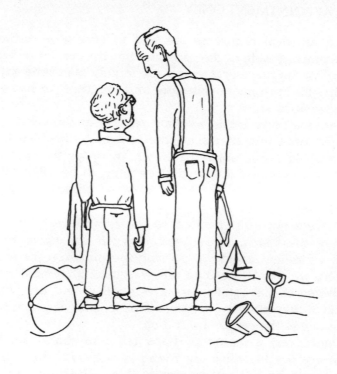

26

The Odd Couple

ONE OF MY very best friends lives and works in the Netherlands. We have known each other since we discovered a mutual interest in herbal medicine and even though we now live on opposite sides of the water, we welcome any opportunity to meet each other. As we are both interested and actively involved in complementary medicine, we sometimes meet at conferences abroad and on one particular occasion this was the case in Portugal.

I have said already that we would make the most of any opportunity to get together, and here we were presented with an ideal chance as we had to choose a partner for the practical side of the seminar. So, the two of us teamed up. The language problems were largely overcome with the help of a Portuguese colleague and together we had a very enjoyable time.

After a fairly hectic working session at the clinic, which lasted until mid-afternoon, the two of us decided to take a relaxing stroll along the beach in order to wind down before a working dinner that evening to be followed by a presentation.

If you can, please use your imagination here. Firstly, we were not quite dressed in the typical gear for a stroll along the beach, as we had just left the clinic and not for a moment could we possibly be mistaken for tourists. There we were, threading our way through sunbathers and children at play, still wearing our collars and ties with our jackets draped over our arms. This in itself was a sufficient contrast to the people around us.

Moreover, I should perhaps tell you that I am below average height, while my friend is very tall. He is, in fact, well over six feet and extremely thin, which only serves to accentuate his height. So, whenever we walk together I have to look up to him as we talk, while he has to stoop down to hear me. This was all the more necessary on that Portuguese beach because of the sound of the surf and the general buzz of the crowd.

Of course, our conversation took place in Dutch, although my friend is equally well versed in English, but as Dutch is our mother tongue that is the language we instinctively use.

Suddenly, we heard a loud English voice behind us: "Wow, have you ever seen such an ugly pair?"

Let me assure you that we never turned around to see who had uttered these words, but with a rather undignified smirk, we continued to amble along. In no way did it dampen our appreciation of each other's company!

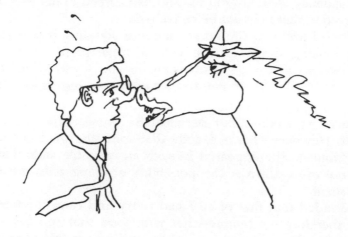

27

Horse Sense

AN ACQUAINTANCE OF mine once asked me to do her a
great favour and have a look at a horse that belonged to a
good friend of hers. It appeared that the horse had recently
become very ill-tempered, which was totally out of character. All of a sudden the horse had become unmanageable
and the owner could not cope with her tantrums. She
had become quite vicious and the veterinary surgeon had
actually advised her to have the horse put down. This, of
course, broke the owner's heart, as she had greatly enjoyed
riding the mare before it had become impossible for anyone

to mount her because she was uncontrollable.

The owner could not make herself accept the drastic solution the vet had offered until she had tried everything possible. She suspected that the reason for the tantrums was jealousy of another horse and had agreed to her friend's suggestion that I should be consulted.

When I first saw the horse, she was standing in a horse-box, looking down on me with a supercilious sneer on her face, as if to say, "And what do you want?" She was indeed a beautiful animal and I could well understand the owner's reluctance to have her put down, not only from the financial viewpoint, but because the horse showed great spirit. However, it was exactly that spirit that had got her into trouble. She appeared in such an excitable state that I did not even consider the possibility of using acupuncture treatment.

I decided that first of all I had to try and calm the horse and therefore we tempted her with food that concealed a homoeopathic tranquilliser. While waiting for this sedative to take effect, I spoke with the owner to try and find out as much as possible about the horse. My first question concerned its diet, and even as I spoke the horse started to neigh loudly, which in turn sent the owner into fits of barely controlled laughter.

I realised that she was very tense as so much was at stake. However, the horse continued to neigh persistently, and this sound was interspersed with sounds of breaking wind. The embarrassed owner tried to reassure me in between her giggles that the horse received the best food that money could buy. Nevertheless, when we discussed the mare's diet in detail, I realised that it was unbalanced and pointed this out to the owner.

Between us, we worked out a new dietary schedule for the horse and the owner could not believe it when within the space of only one week, the horse's behaviour began to change considerably for the better. Of course, after having been so out of sorts and having been allowed to get away with "horse play" for quite some time, the horse had to be retrained and shown who was the boss. Even so, it certainly was not long before she could be ridden again.

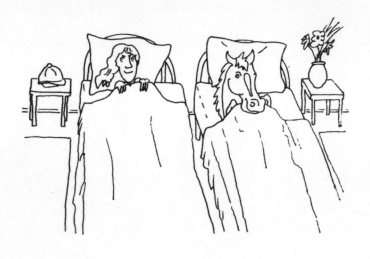

28

Champions

DURING SOME CROSS-COUNTRY horse trials that were
held in our part of the world, a well-known combination
of horse and rider had come to grief at one of the obsta-
cles and both had been injured. The verdict of the veterinary expert was that the horse needed a lengthy period to
recover, and the rider would also be unable to compete for
some time to come. The rider-owner came to me for advice
and treatment and fortunately she responded well.

She then pleaded with me to advise her on her horse
and see if I could do anything for him. The rider was

particularly anxious as she had been training hard and had been selected for an international competition to be held abroad in a fortnight's time. She had pinned all her hopes on that event, as it was of considerable importance to her equestrian career. I did as she asked and both the horse and the rider progressed well on the treatment I decided on. With my approval, the rider then decided to take part in the international event as planned.

I am now the proud owner of a saddle cloth used by that horse during the international trials, at which my two patients proved to be the winning combination. That saddle cloth, together with a note of thanks from the rider, now hangs framed on one of the walls at the clinic and many a time when I pass this arrangement I think back to the gratitude of the rider when she returned to present me with my souvenir. Both rider and horse had overcome their injuries against all the odds in such a short time that they once again proved themselves winners.

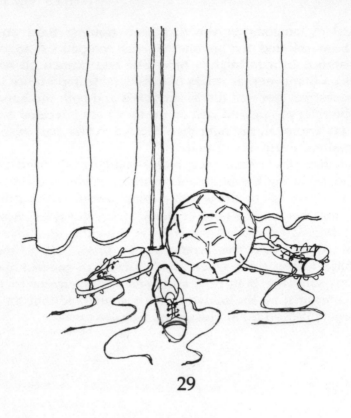

29

Sporting Rivals

ONCE, AFTER A particularly gruelling football match, five Glasgow Celtic players were sent to our clinic for treatment. I knew the boys well enough on an individual basis, as they were fairly regular patients, but this time I had five of them undergoing treatment — all at the same time. They had an important match ahead of them and would need all their wits, fitness and stamina and there was an atmosphere of general excitement. They were looking forward to their next confrontation, which happened to be against their rivals from the same city, namely Rangers.

I moved around between the cubicles while I gave manipulation to one, massage to another and advice to the next. I never like to see any opportunity wasted where I can advise people on how important diet is for their stamina and mental awareness and so I was in my element dishing out snippets of information and suggestions that might help them during their training programme.

Little did I know that one of my colleagues had shown yet another patient into one of the other cubicles for treatment. When I went in to see what was to be done, he said: "Thanks for the good advice, Doc, but I'm sorry to say that I am a Rangers player."

On the field they may be rivals, but in the clinic there reigned a good feeling of comradeship. The game in question was won by Celtic on that occasion, but I did not lose my Rangers player as a patient. In fact, he brought a few of his colleagues along the next time he needed treatment.

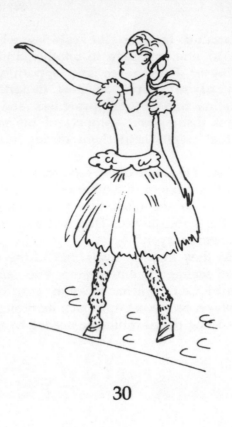

30

The Ballerina

ALONG WITH MANY sports personalities, I have also treated quite a few stage performers, one of them being a ballerina who had come over from Australia for her first visit to Scotland. She was due to perform in an event that could very well be the deciding factor as to whether she would be able to break into the international ballet circuit.

During training she had unfortunately injured her foot and the people with whom she was staying had advised her to come to me for treatment. By this time only a few days remained before the event, so she was most anxious to see if I could help her and explained to me how important this event was to her career. Some tiny bone in her foot had become dislodged and in order to rectify this I had to manipulate her foot and ankle. Sadly enough, there was also considerable bruising and swelling around the injury.

After the manipulative treatment I gave her an embrocation and instructed her on how to use it. I should perhaps explain that there are two kinds of embrocation or liniment, one for humans and another for animals. Generally, however, I prefer to work with the embrocation intended for use with animals, because I have seen such marvellous results, especially with the fragile joints and ligaments of horses. I had, however, omitted to point this out to the ballerina.

Armed with my instructions and this particular embrocation she left the clinic, but returned within a quarter of an hour. As she was departing from the premises, she had told her friend who had kindly offered to drive her there about the treatment and the remedy she was to use. She then produced the liniment out of her bag while travelling in the car and proceeded to read the instructions on the packaging. It was then that she realised that what I had asked her to use was an embrocation for horses. Immediately, she asked her friend to turn the car round and head straight back to the clinic.

When I passed through the reception area she stopped me, waving the remedy about and asked me in a distressed voice, "Dr de Vries, do I look like a horse to you?"

I apologised for my oversight in not explaining to her that I had great faith in that particular remedy or I would not have given it to her, as I also wanted her to do well.

No doubt my happiness cannot have matched hers when I received a large bouquet of flowers a few days later with the message that her performance had gone extremely well and she had been given the part she had coveted. She commented in her note that it was possible that her recovery was due to the manipulative treatment, but she preferred to think that it was as a result of the recommended horse remedy!

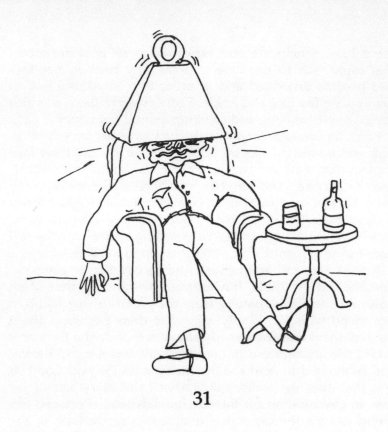

31

Old Habits Die Hard

ONE DAY, ON my way to the treatment-room, I noticed a gentleman in the reception area who was banging his head against the wall at regular intervals. He looked to be in great distress and when I led him into the consulting-room, he told me that he was going out of his mind because of his unbearable migraines. He was desperate and did not know where to turn: all the recommendations and treatments he had received from the various doctors he had approached had brought no change to his condition and he had appeared at our clinic because his general practitioner had finally suggested that acupuncture treatment might possibly bring relief.

We discussed his medical history and his dietary habits and I advised him on some dietary changes he should make, before giving him some remedies and taking him through for his acupuncture treatment. Some time later, he returned for his next appointment and informed me that there had been no improvement in the frequency or severity of his headaches. Again, we discussed the various instructions I had given him and he was given a further session of acupuncture treatment.

When he turned up for the third time with the disappointing news that his condition still remained unchanged, I more or less told him that we would have one last try. If he still experienced no relief, then it was fairly obvious that I was unable to help him and he might as well save himself the trouble of travelling to our clinic as well as the money for the treatment. Moreover, I would then be able to concentrate on those patients whom I was able to help.

However, I felt extremely sorry for him, as well as frustrated, because I find failure hard to swallow, so when I discovered that his wife had accompanied him for his appointment I invited her to join us in the consulting-room.

Between the three of us we went over the various instructions and recommendations yet again and he certainly came across as being totally co-operative. His wife, however, pointed out that there was one little piece of advice that he had not heeded. I was told that he was a docker and every day on his way home from work he stopped off at the pub, where he usually ordered a double whisky — this was his way of unwinding. As he saw no harm in that, he had not changed his habit because he considered that it relaxed him. He thought that without this relaxation his migraines might very well become worse.

From an iridology test I had conducted earlier I had already diagnosed a liver problem and this had been confirmed during acupuncture treatment. He admitted that he had not told me this for fear of being instructed to break the habit of which he was so fond. Fortunately, I managed to persuade him to give my advice a try and not take alcohol for the next month. I also prescribed him a specific remedy for his liver.

When he came back to see me for his next appointment he claimed that the new prescription was fantastic as he had been more or less free from migraines and he felt better than he had for a long, long time. Tongue in cheek, I told him that the remedy may have played a part, but I was convinced that the major benefit had been obtained from the fact that he had gone "on the wagon".

The choice was his now and I spelled out the two options to him: he could either continue his daily indulgence of a double whisky and consequently continue to suffer the interminable migraines, or he could decide to forego his daily drink and benefit from a better quality of life.

He agreed that the choice was simple. He reckoned that it was a small price to pay for a life free from those dreaded migraine attacks and we both considered that case solved. I have met him once or twice since, when he expressed his gratitude yet again and certainly several new patients have informed me that they had been persuaded to make an appointment to see me as a result of speaking with him.

Then, one day, a lady was shown into my consulting-room who was half bent over with back trouble. I discovered that she had "slipped a disc" and took her through to the treatment-room. During the ensuing treatment I managed to relieve the pressure on her sciatic nerve and she then proceeded to lower herself off the treatment-bench without any help from me. I told her what I expected her to do and that she would soon be her old self again if she took care.

This lady told me that she worked as a barmaid and that her boss had been to our clinic for treatment and had strongly recommended that she come to see me for her back problems. Not only had her boss recommended me, but also one of the regulars. Well, he was a regular of a kind. He used to come in every day, in fact, and then she had not seen him for a long time. Recently, however, he had turned up again for an occasional drink. Seemingly, he had been to see me about his migraines and I had worked wonders for him. So, I could not have come with better recommendations, she told me.

This lady departed in a happy frame of mind, but her enthusiastic chatter left me feeling rather disturbed. My suspicions were aroused and, indeed, not long afterwards I saw my patient with the migraines sitting in the waiting-room, banging his head against the wall yet again.

When he entered the consulting-room, I told him that I knew why he was back and scornfully he asked if I counted clairvoyance among my many talents. I told him that I also knew why his headaches were back. Miserably, he confessed that he had not been able to break the old habit and had occasionally imbibed without paying too high a price. Then before he knew it, these migraines had become part of his daily life once more.

This time he cured himself. Every now and then we meet by chance, or I hear about him from other patients, and I hear his problems have not recurred. He has realised that in his case alcohol acts like a poison to his system and that he has no alternative but to avoid it.

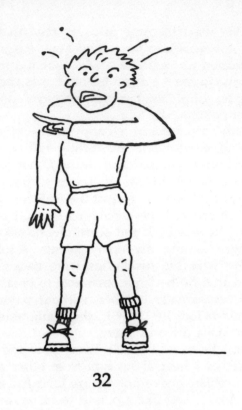

32

Infantile Imagination

A YOUNG MOTHER, accompanied by a little toddler, had been shown into the consulting-room. She, too, was seeking my help as she suffered badly from headaches. She explained that she had been forced to bring her son along as he was too young to be left on his own and she had not been able to find anyone to take care of him.

After I had examined her, I told her that she needed manipulative treatment for a neck adjustment and asked her to follow me to the treatment-room. She took her son by the hand and when we had entered the treatment-room she lay down on a couch and told her son to stay by her side. While I was manipulating her spine and neck, her son suddenly took off. He ran into the crowded waiting-room, where he shouted loudly, amidst great hilarity mixed with some consternation: "That man is taking ma Ma's heid off!"

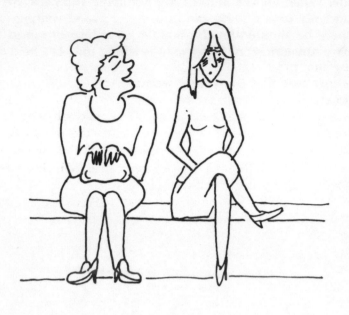

33

Chitchat

EVEN IN THE dentist's waiting-room one can often over-
hear particulars of a patient's medical history being discussed by those waiting to go in for treatment. My wife
assures me that the worst places for such conversations are
the waiting-rooms of ante-natal clinics. All the ins and outs
of childbirth are discussed and the unfortunate first-time
mother-to-be could very easily be put off and frightened
by all the detailed and graphic descriptions of someone
else's experiences. As with waiting-rooms in all medical
establishments, ours is no different. Even when one is

not that way inclined, sometimes not wanting to be rude, one feels obliged to respond to the enquiries of a curious neighbour.

One young female patient, much to her embarrassment, was pressed for information about the nature of her ailment by her nosy, elderly neighbour. The receptionist told me afterwards that the young woman had unsuccessfully tried to avoid mentioning the reason for her visit. Finally she had whispered that she was consulting me about her infertility. The older lady seemed not to recognise the word and asked her to repeat it, which the younger of the two did. The nosy patient then stated in a loud voice: "Oh, it's infertility you're seeing him about then, is it?"

At this point the younger woman looked as if she wished the floor to open up and swallow her, while the general reaction in the waiting-room was mixed. Most people were mildly amused, but the older generation clearly did not think much of this intrusion into one's privacy. The interviewer, however, remained totally oblivious to the fact that she had deeply embarrassed her young neighbour and continued talking away with the greatest of ease.

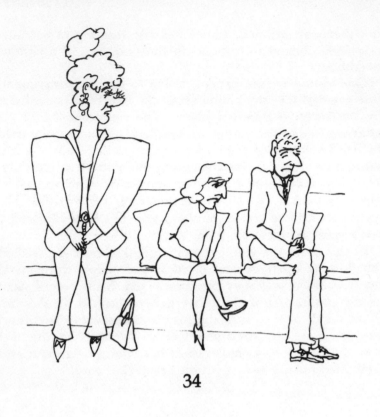

34

A Useful Tip

PASSING THROUGH THE reception area one day, I recognised a lady who was a regular patient at the clinic. Her teenage daughter was seated next to her and her husband sat two chairs away as those in between were occupied. They were a local family, quite well-to-do but with airs and graces above their station. The mother was very hard of hearing, but refused to wear a hearing-aid out of misplaced pride. Whenever the mother had an appointment at the clinic, all three of them would arrive together, as the father was needed to drive.

The lady in question was fashionably turned out in a well-cut pair of trousers with a matching jacket. Her daughter had obviously realised that her mother's zip was undone and pointed this out to her in a low voice.

The mother asked loudly, "Who wants a tip?"

The daughter repeated to the mother, "Your zip, Mother."

"Tip? Who am I supposed to tip?" replied the mother querulously.

The daughter then reiterated crossly and loudly, "Your zip is open, Mother!" and pointed to the offending object.

The mother calmly put down her handbag, stood up and with her nose in the air, proceeded to pull up her zip.

I could not help noticing her husband at this point, cringing in his chair and trying to look as if they did not belong together.

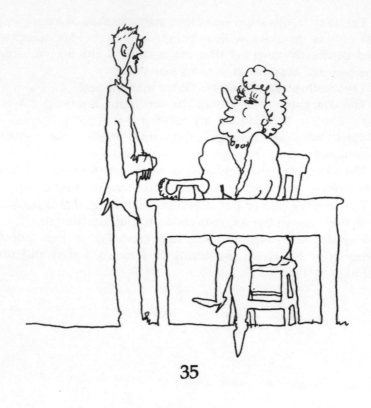

35

A Matter of Etiquette

AT A SOCIAL function I made the acquaintance of a gentleman who was introduced to me as the Duke of X. He took advantage of this introduction to ask me for a consultation. When I returned to the clinic, I asked my receptionist to make a note of his appointment in the appointment book. Shortly afterwards, I received a telephone call from him asking me if it would be possible for him to bring along a friend, the Duke of Z, as he also wanted to consult me. As they were planning to travel together, I agreed.

When I asked my receptionist to amend the appointment

book accordingly, she asked me how she was supposed to address them. Mrs Beaton's book on etiquette was duly consulted, in which it was discovered that they ought to be addressed as "Your Grace".

Shortly before the time arranged for their appointment, in walked a gentleman who gave his name at the desk as the Duke of X, and indeed my receptionist remembered to address him as "Your Grace". He then went on to inform her that, unfortunately, his friend the Duke of Z had not been able to keep his appointment and sent his apologies. My receptionist must have become slightly flustered at this point, because she looked up at him and said, "I'll make a note of that — and in the meantime would you like to take a seat please, Duke dear?"

Fortunately the Duke joined in the general outburst of laughter, while my receptionist swallowed deeply and stared at him, her cheeks scarlet with embarrassment, as she realised what she had said. Afterwards, the Duke told me that he had been addressed in many ways, but never before as "Duke dear"!

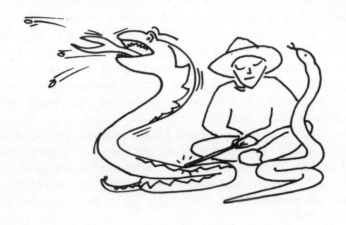

36

A Bizarre Experience

DURING MY TIME in China I once found myself queueing in a street market. I had been troubled with a persistent stomach upset, most likely because something I had eaten had disagreed with me. Anyway, I had been told to go to this market, where I would find, on the right-hand side, a stall from which I could obtain some snake poison. This, I had been told, would definitely sort out my stomach problems.

I can tell you that I stood there for some time, fascinated by the bustling activity around me. You name it, and it was for sale there: vegetables, fish, poultry, meat, trinkets, clothes, songbirds — everything you can think of. There were even grimy stalls where pieces of meat, fowl, snake or fish were thrown into large vats of boiling oil. These delicacies were then ladled on to newspaper and offered for immediate consumption. I was mesmerised by all these new experiences.

The queue for the stall selling snake poison was long, but as there was so much to see I had no chance to become bored. As I inched forward, I finally had a chance to see what was happening. Beside the stall an elderly woman sat on a low stool. On either side of her were a number of jute or burlap sacks, which convulsed every now and then with the movement of the snakes held captive inside.

I personally had never worked with snake poison before, but had certainly heard plenty of good reports about its efficacy from those who had.

For those who are unfamiliar with the subject, perhaps a very brief explanation of the homoeopathic principles is in order here. Dr Hahnemann, the founder of homoeopathy, followed Parcelsus' principle *"Similia Similiabus Curetur"*, i.e. "Like Cures Like". Homoeopathic remedies are basically diluted solutions, the strength of which varies between 30:1 and 100:1, the latter obviously being a weaker potency.

Snake poison is supposed to work on a similar principle to that of homoeopathy and by doing so would therefore fit nicely into complementary medicine as a whole.

Returning to my story, however, when I got near enough to the stall to be able to see exactly what was happening, I smartly removed myself from the queue. The old woman was sitting there, skinning snakes and removing their entrails. These were then wrapped up in a paper and sold for use as an aphrodisiac. When snake poison was requested, on the other hand, the old woman would grip a snake by the head and briefly touch it with a red-hot-poker on its cervical vertebrae. The snake, understandably, would react furiously to this and spit out its venom, which in turn was skilfully caught in a glass. The contents of this glass would then be diluted with mineral water and offered to the customer who had requested it. That customer would drink that concoction on the spot.

I noticed that the cobra seemed to be the favourite snake for this purpose, although the old lady did extract venom from other species as well. But not being a connoisseur of snakes, I could not tell you their names.

Possibly you may think that I am too soft-hearted, but I hate to see pain inflicted on any creature and even though I am not at all fond of snakes, this red-hot poker treatment was more than I could bear to watch. I quickly gave up my place in the queue, which of course left me with the predicament that I still had not obtained the homoeopathic solution I had waited for so patiently in order to settle my stomach disorder.

Instead, I went to a hospital clinic, where I found a doctor who spoke good English and explained the situation to him. He smiled indulgently and took a bottle from the medicine cupboard and poured some of its contents into a glass. This he handed to me to drink and as I did so he stood and watched me with typical Chinese inscrutability. When I had taken the medicine he assured me that my stomach problems would be solved by tomorrow. I then enquired as to what he had just given me, only to learn that it was exactly the same remedy as the one I had queued for in the market.

To give him his due, he was right; by the following morning my stomach problems had indeed disappeared!

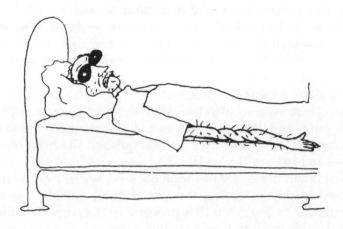

37

Who Was the Victim?

THE EVENT I will recount below was not actually experienced by myself, but by one of my colleagues. You will understand what it is like during conferences or seminars. All kinds of unusual cases are discussed among us and this incident was so out of the ordinary that it has stayed in my memory.

My colleague has a busy practice in the centre of a large city. One evening, after a hectic surgery, he was in the process of locking up the premises and looking forward to getting home as quickly as possible. Suddenly, he was attacked by two young men. One of them grabbed him from the back and held his neck in an armhold, while the other immediately went for the inside pocket of his jacket and pulled out his wallet.

Fortunately, this colleague happens to be a very accomplished osteopath. I say "fortunately" because he kept his wits about him and as the second assailant pulled the wallet from his pocket, my colleague grabbed his wrist and twisted it. A twist is quite an ordinary movement in osteopathy. However, under normal circumstances the movement is used to put some joint *into* place, rather than *out* of place, as was the case here.

The twist was so effective that the young man writhed with pain and then passed out. This alarmed the other assailant to the extent that he relinquished his hold on the victim and took to his heels.

First of all, my colleague took back his wallet and then re-entered his clinic leaving the victim lying outside. He was determined to deal with this problem in the correct manner. First he phoned the police and reported the attempted robbery and then he phoned for an ambulance. The police duly arrived, as did the ambulance, and my colleague saw that the young man was laid on a stretcher and taken off to hospital for treatment. He was then interviewed by the police, who made a preliminary report and informed him that he was free to go home. They told him that they would be back the next day, when a more detailed report would be prepared on the basis of which it would be decided what action would be taken.

My colleague finally arrived home considerably later than anticipated and he had barely started telling his wife about his unfortunate experience, when the phone rang. His wife took the call and informed her husband that a hospital doctor wanted to speak to him. He went to the phone, only to hear from the doctor in question that he had been attending to the young man with the twisted wrist. The patient had by this time regained consciousness, but was still in great pain. The doctor, it transpired, was not sure how to deal with the twisted joint and was therefore phoning my colleague to ask him if he would be so kind as to come to the hospital and give the young man the required treatment.

My colleague made his way to the hospital and spoke to the young man. He said that he would help him, but only on condition that the young man promised never to take part in such an assault again. The promise was given, and my colleague proceeded to treat the young man.

Obviously, my colleague cannot be sure whether the promise has been honoured, but let us hope that the young man has learned a lesson from his experience!

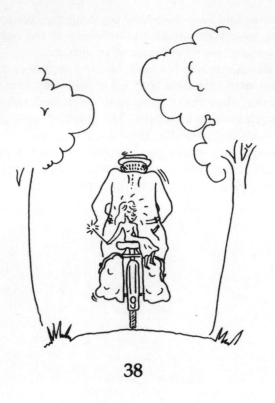

38

A Fairy Tale

I HAVE ALREADY pointed out that part of the reason why I opted to run a day clinic rather than the residential clinic was the fact that with the latter we were so heavily dependent on reliable staff. With our present clinic we are not quite as badly handicapped if one or two members of staff fail to turn up for work without prior notice. Naturally, the smooth running of the clinic is affected, but other arrangements can be made at short notice. This always seemed to be more difficult with the residential clinic.

Anyway, I consider myself to have been lucky with the

staff I have employed over the years, as they have mostly proven to be dependable and trustworthy. There again, we have also had our disappointing moments, of which the following incident is one.

One day my dietician asked for a few moments of my time as she wished to discuss a rather delicate problem with me. According to her, a number of items from the store-room had been mysteriously disappearing. She was not talking about major items, as it appeared that they were everyday groceries that went missing, such as loaves of bread, packets of butter, and fruit. She told me too that initially she had wondered if our deliveries had been short and had therefore made a point of checking them all personally, but found that the fault did not lie with the suppliers.

As our store-room could be approached from the outside it was fairly difficult to keep a close eye on it. This arrangement had purposely been decided on in order to facilitate the deliveries; but now we found that it also had its disadvantages.

Any incident like this puts a damper on the general atmosphere, as everyone feels under suspicion until the culprit has been identified. Furthermore, not only was it a disappointment to learn that there was someone among the staff who could not be trusted, but the additional problem arose that we would sometimes run out of necessities, which caused great embarrassment. Therefore, some of the staff who had been with us for a long time and whom I trusted implicitly, were informed of the matter and asked to keep a look-out.

It was mentioned to me that our handyman had been seen going into the store-room more often that it was felt he had reason to. He used to cycle into work every day on his bicycle with, hanging on either side of the luggage carrier, two sturdy canvas bags. I felt I had no alternative but to check these bags and, sure enough, that afternoon I found several grocery items packed inside that were of the same brand as we had in our store-room. I did not consider this in itself to be sufficient evidence with which to confront him and therefore I decided on another tactic. I mentioned to him that a certain amount of pilfering had been discovered and asked for his assistance in keeping an eye on the store-room. If he saw anything untoward, would he please let me know. This he promised readily and also told me that the guilty person deserved to be penalised severely, as this was no way to repay my trust.

During the next two days the pilfering continued as before, and again I saw familiar items in the bags on his bicycle. I decided to give him one last chance before confronting him with my suspicions and I asked him if he had come up with anything that could solve the puzzle of the disappearing groceries. He replied that he had no idea who the culprit might be; he had, however, been wondering if possibly the fairies might be to blame.

I was astounded to hear this and asked him if he was being serious. He then said that he couldn't think of anyone else. Looking him straight in the eye, I told him that to my way of thinking he could well be that fairy and as he had been so insistent on the severity of the punishment that had to be meted out, what penalty did he have in mind for himself? At least he had the decency to finally admit to the pilfering. He told me that he had to support a large family and pleaded with me not to make a formal complaint against him and to keep the police out of the matter. If I agreed, he said, he would punish himself in the worst possible way he could imagine: he would dismiss himself from our employment and I would never see him again.

True enough, he kept his word. From that day on I never saw nor heard of him again. Unfortunately, we later realised that items more valuable than simple groceries had also disappeared, but we had to put that down to experience as well!

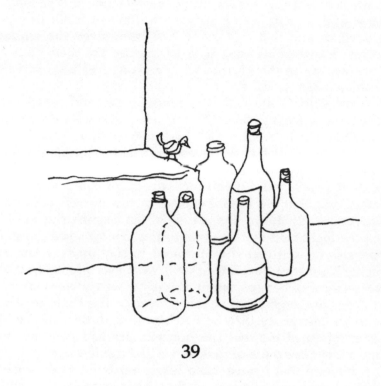

39

A Shortage of Pintas

WE HAD FINALLY been able to fill the vacancy for a housekeeper and this was making life considerably easier for us. The lady who had taken over that function had presented us with good references and she appeared to be a pleasant and reliable person. After the initial period of settling in and coming to grips with her job, we all became accustomed to the new routine.

However, one thing slightly puzzled me about her; occasionally, but not always, she seemed to be somewhat preoccupied and absent-minded. Then, one day, there was great

115

confusion and a general unhappiness among the patients. Most of them had been instructed to follow specific dietary guidelines and that day many had been given the wrong meals. I know how easy it is to confuse the diets of two patients, but in this case nearly everyone had been served with incorrect meals.

I raised the issue with the housekeeper and asked her if she was feeling unwell or if she was worried about possible health problems. I had noticed that she drank large amounts of liquid, particularly milk, so I considered it a possibility that she might be diabetic. No, she felt perfectly well and I need not worry. It was, however, rather odd that we often seemed to run out of milk and that frequently during the course of the evening she would tell the night staff that she had to pop out for some more. I had also noticed that she appeared to stay up very late at night. No matter how late it was, whenever I looked up at the window of her apartment, the lights were always on.

Then, one night, I was called over to the clinic to deal with an emergency. After I had attended to this, the night sister informed me that the housekeeper had gone out to buy a few more pints of milk as we had run low again.

I am sure that I must have taken her by surprise when she returned, but she was really too far gone for it to sink in. She walked into the clinic and, apart from hearing her singing away to herself, I immediately noticed that her hat was perched on her head back to front. I told her to take herself off to bed and added that I wanted to speak to her the following morning.

At breakfast the next day she went about her duties as usual and made no reference whatsoever to the previous evening. When I called her into the office and asked her if she had packed her bags, she looked at me in total surprise. I had to remind her of what I had witnessed the previous evening and pointed out to her that despite several offers of help, she had remained adamant that there was nothing wrong. Considering the responsibility she carried

116

with the function of housekeeper, I concluded, it would be impossible for me to keep her on in that capacity.

Whatever kind of pints she takes at present is not known to me, but for her sake I hope that she sticks to the milk. Somehow, however, I doubt it!

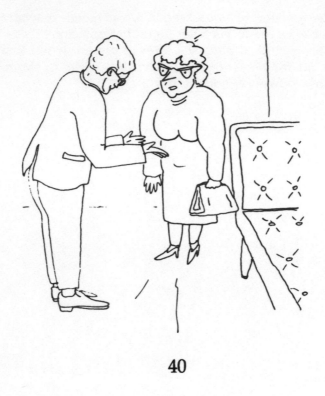

40

Language Lessons

EVEN WHEN ONE has learned to converse fairly comfortably in another language, there are always surprises in store. Our daughters were born in the Netherlands, but they were still quite young when my wife and I decided to move to Scotland and start a practice there. My wife, being Scottish, was in fact returning home, but although I had visited Scotland often enough, I had never actually lived there. I have said before, never once have I regretted that decision to move to Scotland. The whole family was bilingual, so few problems were envisaged in that respect.

Although my English was good enough to get by, I did not have a strong grasp of colloquialisms. Nevertheless, one learns as one goes along. That was certainly the case with me, although at times I have been greatly puzzled by certain Scottish expressions.

During my first week of practice I was consulted by a patient who had been referred to me by her general practitioner for back problems. She was a pleasant middle-aged lady and was married to a farmer. In order to reach a correct diagnosis I had to examine her and asked her to remove her outer garments. She did not respond and looked at me blankly. So, I repeated my request for her to take off all her clothes except her underwear. Hesitantly she queried, "Ye mean A've tae tak aff ma claish?"

As the last word was slightly reminiscent of the Dutch word for clothes, I nodded. We seemed to have understood each other as she indeed took off her dress. She stood there looking at me expectantly and I asked her to also remove her vest. Again she looked at me blankly and I therefore pointed to her vest and repeated my request. With a broad smile she responded, "That's no a vest, that's ma semmit!" So, that was yet another word I could add to my growing vocabulary.

I proceeded with her treatment and massaged and manipulated the patient's spine. At one stage during the session I asked her to sit up straight. Asking for confirmation she turned her head towards me and said, "Ye want me tae sit on ma bum?" I understood the last word to be the equivalent of her posterior, so again I agreed and I must have been correct, because she moved to the required position. The treatment was completed without any further confusion or guessing games.

In common with many foreigners, I also have the tendency to remember the wrong words. Therefore it may not surprise you that for some time afterwards I continued to ask my patients to please sit on their bums — and they would oblige. Never for a moment did I realise that this was incorrect English. It was not until my wife heard me use the word to one of our children that she remarked on my growing vocabulary and when I told her that this was one of the few words I had learned from the farmer's wife, and that it stood me in good stead in my work, she could no longer contain herself. Gleefully, she explained to me that it was not only a word used in Scottish dialect, but also a colloquialism in the English language with the same meaning, but that it definitely did not belong in a doctor's vocabulary!

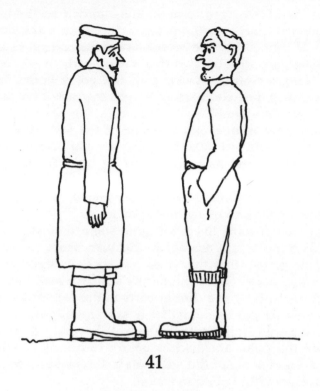

41

The Better Deal

AN ELDERLY FARMER was a regular patient at the clinic. His limbs had grown very stiff, undoubtedly as a result of his working outdoors in all kinds of weather. His knees especially plagued him and he happily turned up for regular acupuncture treatment, as he claimed that this was the only thing that helped to keep him on his feet and therefore enable him to continue running his farm.

One late afternoon he turned up for his appointment as usual. It had been one of those days that are best forgotten: the waiting-room had been crowded all day long and no sooner had I managed to make some inroad on the backlog of patients, than something seemed to disrupt the flow yet again. It seemed to have been a day of fits and starts and, to be honest, we were all glad that it was nearly over. We were all looking forward to locking up and going home, hoping that the next day would bring fewer surprises of the kind we could well do without.

The farmer in question was one of the last patients that day. His treatment was basically straightforward and he knew the routine as well as any of us. We had grown quite friendly over the years and always managed to have a little chat. This time, however, he treated us to a yarn that brightened the end of a ghastly day for us.

Now that I have lived for quite some time in Scotland, I have come to appreciate the Scottish sense of humour, but I do realise that this does not apply to everyone. For example, I once related the farmer's story which I am going to tell you shortly at a dinner party in the Netherlands. One of the dinner guests immediately saw the humour of it, but then she was from Scottish descent. Several others totally missed the point and had to ask for clarification, which of course takes some of the shine off it. Possibly my rendering had lost something in translation.

Anyway, the farmer was shown into the treatment-room and as he was making himself comfortable on the couch, he exclaimed that the most unusual thing had happened to him that day and chuckled to himself. As he spoke in quite a strong Scottish brogue, I will not even try to emulate this on paper, even though it would bring the story to life.

He told me that he had had the most extraordinary meeting with a cattle dealer. Filling me in on the background, he explained that he had bought two calves from the dealer on market day, three weeks previously. He had been happy enough with his purchase and had taken the calves home and seen to it that they were well taken care of. Unfortunately, within the first week both calves had died and on market day the following week he told some of his friends about his misfortune over a pint in the pub.

His friends asked him what he was going to say to the dealer who had sold him the calves when they met again. The farmer explained that he was going to let the matter rest because his losses had been covered by insurance, but he would certainly think twice before having any dealings with that particular dealer again.

By a stroke of luck, as he was leaving the bank later that afternoon after attending to some business, he spotted the dealer walking down the road. He crossed the street to speak to the man and informed him that the calves he had bought from him three weeks ago had both died within one week. The dealer looked at him for a second or two, as if deciding what to say. Then he took the farmer's hand and, while pumping this up and down, he congratulated him.

No other response could have surprised the farmer more. He stared at the dealer and muttered something about why were congratulations considered to be in order, because, for goodness sake, his two calves were dead!

The dealer then explained that on that same day he had also sold two calves to another farmer and as far as he knew those two calves were still alive. My friend, the farmer, totally nonplussed by this, blurted out that he did not care for the other farmer's calves because his own two were dead. It was then the dealer piped up with the response that he ought to consider himself lucky, because the other chap's calves were still alive, but the farmer himself was dead!

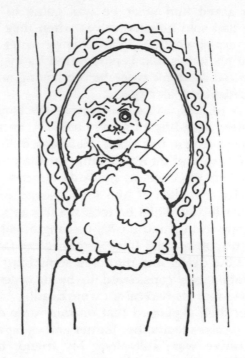

42

A Migraine Cure

ONE OF MY regular patients was a lady who suffered frequently from migraines. This problem was largely brought about by fairly advanced glaucoma in one eye. Before she ever came to our clinic, her other eye had been so badly affected by this disease that it had to be removed, and in its place she had been fitted with an artificial eye.

We had tried several therapies for her migraines, but from experience it appeared that acupuncture treatment gave her the best results. This was despite the fact that she made no bones about not being very keen on the treatment.

One day, however, when she turned up for her appointment she told me, giggling, that she had now discovered the most comfortable and pleasant treatment for a migraine attack and challenged me to do the worst with my acupuncture needles, because she really was not bothered. It seemed to me that she was speaking in riddles and so I asked her to explain herself. She looked at me with a twinkle in her remaining eye and then made herself comfortable before recounting her story in great detail.

Still with a huge smile on her face, she told me that the previous day she had felt a migraine attack coming on and had decided to lie down for a few hours in the afternoon. As her artificial eye sometimes irritated her during a migraine attack, she had removed it and placed it on her bedside table.

She had not been lying down for long when she heard the doorbell ring and so she decided to ignore it. However, the bell was rung a second time and her peace was shattered when she contemplated that it could be something urgent. She swung her legs out and in the darkened room groped about for her glass eye and pushed it in position while making her way to the door, meanwhile running her hands quickly through her hair to smarten herself up. She opened the door to find two gentlemen, who gave her one look and immediately took to their heels. Surprised by this, and somewhat annoyed at the unwelcome intrusion, she closed the door and decided to forget about having a rest.

Still giggling away to herself while relating this story in beautiful detail, she went on to tell me that she had gone back to the bedroom to open the curtains and when she had turned towards the dressing-table to run a comb through her hair, she had caught sight of herself in the mirror and immediately understood what had sent the two gentlemen running off. In her hurry to answer the door, she had just "plonked" in her artificial eye and now she realised she had put it in back to front. The white of the back of the eye was staring at her from the mirror and she had burst out laughing when she saw what she looked like. She admitted that she herself thought that she presented a frightful sight and howled with laughter.

She removed the eye and put it back correctly, but before she had managed to control her laughter the doorbell rang again. Once more she answered the door, only to find the same two gentlemen on the doorstep. They had returned to apologise for their bad manners and to find out if she was all right.

They explained that they were representatives of a certain religious group and had called on the off-chance to talk to her, but taking account of her migraine they would leave her in peace for now and call back some other time.

She finished her story by telling me that when the gentlemen had disappeared she had sat down in a chair and had a jolly good laugh about it all and came to the conclusion that at some time during all the carry-on her migraine had totally disappeared, which only goes to show that laughter can be a great healer!

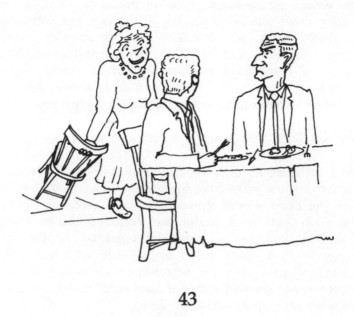

43

Bad Form

IT ALWAYS CREATES somewhat of a dilemma if I meet patients from home when I am on my travels. They often seem to act as if they own me and I cannot quite make out if they think they have this right because we are neither of us on home territory. What I do know, however, is that it can be extremely embarrassing.

Usually my travels abroad take place because I have been invited to attend some conference or seminar. In those instances my time is very precious and, in common with other practitioners, I too welcome the opportunity to renew my friendships with colleagues whom I hardly ever meet except on such occasions. We generally arrange to meet up, in groups of two or more, with people whom we consider to be on the same wave-length and who share similar interests. If we are specialists in each other's fields, we also take this opportunity to put our heads together and discuss new developments. This exchange of knowledge is very important because new ideas and information stream in from all over the world at such events. Although the formal lectures are very interesting and helpful, it is often the case that more can be learned from speaking to colleagues on a one-to-one basis.

I once attended an international conference in Spain and, like most of those attending the congress, I was booked to stay in the hotel where the conference was being held. I had met up with an acquaintance from the United States and we had arranged to meet for breakfast on the first morning, to bring each other up to date with the latest developments in a project in which we were both involved. This conference seemed like the ideal opportunity to catch up on what each other had been doing.

We had just placed our order with the waiter when a lady approached our table. She exclaimed loudly that she had spotted me from across the dining room and was delighted to see me because she wanted my advice. I quickly recognised the lady as one of my patients, who, it turned out, happened to be staying in the same hotel for a holiday. I was obliged to introduce her to my colleague and, without having been invited to do so, she promptly pulled up a chair and joined us at our table.

I did not have a chance to inform my friend that this lady happened to be a great hypochondriac with little else to occupy her mind but her extreme anxiety about anything relating to her health and imaginary illnesses. He soon discovered what kind of person we were up against, however, because all during breakfast she dominated the conversation. She was a pleasant enough person in herself, but all her aches and pains had to be aired in the conversation, and she more or less used my colleague to gain confirmation of my diagnosis and then obtain a second opinion on the course of action I had advised.

When the time of our first lecture arrived, we left the dining room, feeling thoroughly downhearted by this lady's bad manners and by what we considered to have been a wasted hour. We therefore decided to meet for an early breakfast the following day, as we both had other commitments for the remainder of that day.

Lo and behold, the next morning this lady must have been lying in wait for us. We had asked the waiter for a quiet table tucked away in a corner, but unfortunately our mistake was to meet so early, before the dining room had a chance to fill up. It was therefore relatively easy for her to spot us.

She once again launched into her tirade, but this time we showed less patience; we informed her, fairly bluntly, that we had a lot of work to get through and asked her would she please be so kind as to leave us to it. We really thought we had cracked it when she left our table.

However, she was more persistent than we had given her credit for, because shortly afterwards she reappeared, complaining about a pain in her knee and asking what I thought she ought to do about it. Having reached the end of his tether, my colleague calmly informed her that he was convinced that she must be suffering from syphilis and that nothing could be done about it. That was it — she rose from the table and indignantly marched off.

My colleague rubbed his hands gleefully and stated that I was well rid of her. Anyway, she did not know him, so it did not matter what he had said — and as for me, I would be better off without her!

Despite the unwelcome interruptions we managed to bring each other up to date before the end of the conference and said our goodbyes before going our separate ways again. Much to my surprise, I received a letter from this lady soon after my return home with the message that she would prefer to cancel her outstanding appointment for the time being because of her disappointment in me — she needed time to consider her association with me in the light of my poor taste in friends!

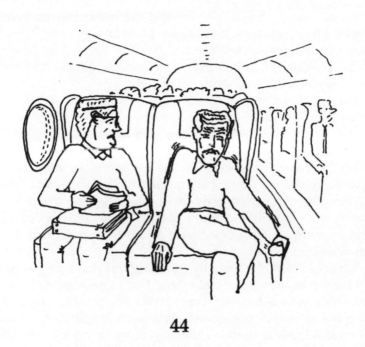

44

A Slight Anticlimax

SOME TIME AGO, when travelling to attend a conference in a neighbouring country, I was sitting in the plane studying my notes when I noticed that the gentleman sitting next to me was shivering all over. He was an elderly gentleman who looked very tense and preoccupied, and I realised that he was extremely upset about something. Even though I wanted to concentrate on my preparations for the conference, I felt that I had to speak to him.

When the general bustle of people finding their seats and stowing away their hand luggage had eased somewhat, I enquired if he was all right. He replied that he would do anything to be allowed to step off the plane again. He had never flown before and he had always turned down his daughter's invitations to visit her. She lived in the country of our destination. Finally, he had succumbed to her entreaties, but really regretted his promise to come over, because he was so afraid of flying.

He explained that, as she was sympathetic to his fear of flying, his daughter had always come over to see him and his wife, but now that she had a young family of her own this was no longer so easy for her. His wife had died recently and as he wanted to see his grandchildren, he just had to travel to them. He had no other immediate family — because they had only ever had the one child — so there was very little option. Even so, he still did not like the thought of flying, as was certainly apparent from his tenseness.

I tried to allay his fears by pointing out that flying is really by far the safest way of travelling, but I immediately realised that this was achieving very little. So, in this instance, I decided that this frightened passenger might benefit from one of the few remedies I usually carry in my pocket. Over the years I have grown into the habit of carrying one or two useful remedies on me and this had already proved helpful on several previous occasions.

As the cabin crew were still busy helping people to settle themselves, I struggled down the aisle to fetch a small cup of water and offered it to my fellow passenger along with the remedy. I assured him that this would ease his tension and that there really was nothing to flying. He would be at his destination before he realised it. By this time he was so uptight that he did not even consider objecting to taking something offered to him by a stranger.

Whether it was to please me, I don't know, but he eased himself as much as possible into his chair, gripped the arm rests and closed his eyes. As all this took place before take-off I couldn't even suggest that he lowered the back of his seat because that would be breaking the rules.

Anyway, he made a great effort to do as was suggested, but I could tell from the way he was gripping the arm rests that he was still struggling for self-control. With his eyes tightly closed and his knuckles white on the arm rests, he breathed deeply. Several minutes passed while the cabin crew made final preparations for the flight.

Eventually, a stewardess gave the usual demonstration concerning escape routes and the use of life-jackets. My fellow passenger had opened his eyes and was listening to this with growing horror, obviously imagining himself deposited in the ocean. I tried to reassure him and urged him to relax, repeating yet again that time passes swiftly in the air and we would arrive at our destination before he knew it. He resumed his deep breathing. All was quiet for a short while. Suddenly, his eyes popped open. Fixing me with a hopeful look, he enquired as to whether, seeing that everything was supposed to go so quietly, we had arrived yet!

Poor man, he was shattered when I had to tell him that we had not yet left the ground!

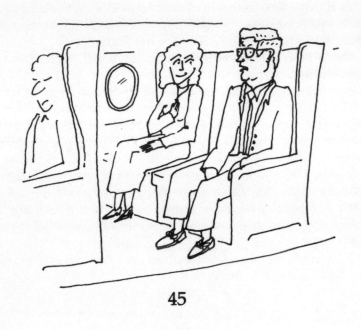

45

Lateral Thinking

THERE ARE ALWAYS two sides to the coin or two ways of looking at a problem. To some people everything is all cut and dried, while others will prevaricate and take their time to come up with a solution or an explanation. Which way is better? The answer to that is anyone's guess, but once I was given a valuable lesson by a quiet young lady.

During a long flight abroad, this lady was seated next to me on the plane. Once or twice during the flight we exchanged pleasantries and she told me that she still had a long journey ahead of her after we had landed. Although she was not wearing a religious habit, I had noticed that she often fingered a large crucifix hanging from a chain around her neck. Therefore I was not surprised when I learned that she had been assigned to a mission and although she was very much looking forward to the work and was happy to be given the chance to put her training to good use, she was rather apprehensive of flying. In fact, this was her very first flight.

With what I considered to be great tact, I pointed out to her that no one would die before their time. Needless to say, I feel that this faith does not exonerate us from acting irresponsibly. Morally we will always remain answerable to our conscience.

The young lady expressed her agreement to this theory, but followed this by a question to which I still have no answer, as I had to admit that I had never before looked at it from that angle. She asked: "Wouldn't it be a pity, though, if it were not yet my time, but that the pilot's time was up?"

135

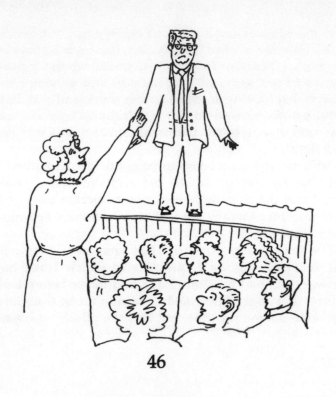

46

A Great Response

NOT SO LONG ago I was invited by one of the Cancer Community Care Centres to give a public talk. This could be a valuable exercise, I thought, as it could serve as an opportunity to clear away some of the misconceptions that seem to be immediately associated with the word "cancer". Until not so very long ago, few people dared even utter the word aloud and would drop their voice to a whisper. "The Big C" was often as far as people dared to go, if they had to give it a name at all.

To many people the subject of cancer unfortunately either brings back sad memories or instills a deep fear.

Because of this dread, the public often has a very limited knowledge of this illness and therefore lacks understanding. It is particularly sad for their friends or relatives who may have been diagnosed as suffering from cancer, because they do not always receive the support they need to face reality. Nowadays, however, the chance of recovery is so very much better than ever before. In fact, quite a few forms of cancer are no longer considered fatal and the sooner this illness is diagnosed and treated, the better chance the patient has of total recovery.

Considering the sensitivity of the subject, I prepared my talk with great care. The organisers had informed me that they expected a good turn-out, as they had received many enquiries.

When the time came, I talked for quite a while on the subject and was impressed by the attention and concentration of the audience. After the talk there was to be an opportunity to ask questions and when we came to that point of the evening, I announced that anyone who would like further explanation on any aspect of my talk was welcome to come forward.

The usual pattern here is that people tend to hold back somewhat. No one actually likes to be the first to speak, just in case other people may consider their question to signify a lack of intelligence. Generally, then, there is a fairly strained silence and sometimes I have to coax the audience gently into the follow-up. But not so this time, however.

Immediately after I had announced that I was now prepared to answer questions, a lady from the second row jumped to her feet. I had noticed her concentration during my address, and not for one minute could I have anticipated her question. I was left speechless! She asked me if I was wearing a wig, and if not, was this my own hair colour or did I have it dyed!

Just imagine how you would feel having such a question thrown at you after having spoken on such a serious subject. I was dumbfounded and wondered how to respond.

Then I thought of my quick visit to the barber's only that afternoon and wondered if she would still have asked me that same question if she had seen me prior to my haircut, when I was sporting an unruly mop of hair.

I have to admit that I was devastated. If that was the best response from an audience I could hope for, I would never waste my breath again by giving public talks. Fortunately, this lady had broken the ice and the calibre of the questions that followed was considerably better.

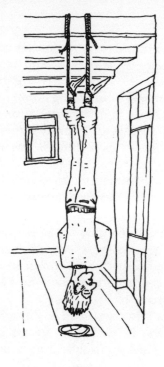

47

Exceptional Credulity

A FEW YEARS ago I wrote a book called *Traditional Home and Herbal Remedies*, which included, together with much useful information, some extremely unusual remedies that I have collected over the years. Grateful patients from the mainland and the islands off the west coast of Scotland had contributed some of their old-fashioned remedies that have been handed down from one generation to the next. I was also given an old diary by a doctor's widow and the collecting of some of these weird and wonderful remedies eventually turned into a joint effort.

I was given descriptions of concoctions that were brewed

from the most extraordinary ingredients. Poultices were also a favourite remedy and these too would contain very unorthodox ingredients. I had many a good laugh with my assistants when we were compiling some of the most bizarre remedies and methods that we came across; in fact many of them we decided to repeat in print largely *because* of their originality. Little did we expect that some people might take them all seriously.

Consider my surprise when I discovered that I had gained a new patient as an unexpected spin-off from this book. A gentleman phoned our clinic to make an appointment concerning his back trouble and when I saw him for his consultation he was near enough bent double. I soon diagnosed a "slipped disc" and enquired if anything out of the ordinary had happened, because he had already told me that he was not prone to back trouble.

It transpired that he had read my book *Traditional Home and Herbal Remedies*, in which he found an old method to cure him of a particular problem he was suffering at the time.

The advice was that if a patient was struck by severe stomach pains, a rope should be put around his feet and then he should be hung by the heels from the rafters. This was to be repeated at regular intervals in order to "undo the knot in the guts". On reflection, he agreed with me that it seemed unwise for anyone to even seriously consider taking such drastic action, but it is easy to be wise after the event.

In fact, my new patient had decided to follow this bizarre piece of advice to the letter and in the process he had badly hurt his back. I gave him full credit, however, for still daring to consult me for his back after conducting such an unfortunate experiment. I am sure that nine out of ten people would have placed me at the bottom of their list of favourite practitioners. Anyway, his back was soon straightened and a few days of taking it easy would put paid to that complaint. For what it was worth, I advised him to do something much less drastic the next time he had stomach pains!

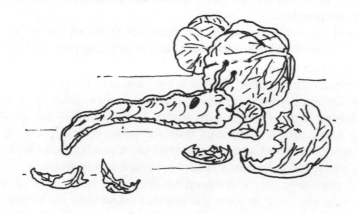

48

Occupational Hazard?

SOME TIME AGO now I spotted a gentleman in the waiting-room who was shivering badly and really looked ill. His face was covered in spots and I noticed that neither seat next to him had been taken by other waiting patients. When he was shown into the consulting-room he told me that he had had this skin condition for quite some time now and that he often felt feverish. Thank goodness, from what he told me I did not feel we were dealing with an infectious disease. He told me that his problems were gradually becoming worse and, apart from the feverish bouts and the general discomfort he experienced, he was very embarrassed about his appearance and certainly had not failed to notice people's hesitancy to be near him.

Seemingly, he had been to see all kinds of doctors and clinics, but no one and nowhere had been able to help him. He had travelled all the way from the south of England to see me, determined to leave no stone unturned. Could I please help him?

I fired one question after the other at him. At times like this I feel more like a detective than a practitioner, but the more a patient tells me, the more likely I am to hit on a clue. That was the case here. He told me that he ran a fairly small nursery, where he grew fruit and vegetables as well as flowers. I questioned him about the chemicals he used in his work and soon found that we were certainly on the right track. A blood test proved that he was allergic to some of the chemical colourings that were used in his work.

Unfortunately, it is frequently the case nowadays that chemicals are used to give the vegetables we see on display at our greengrocer's or supermarket their attractive, vivid colour. This was my patient's downfall.

With his full co-operation a programme was worked out for him. I was able to promise him a full recovery on the understanding that the offending chemicals would have to disappear from his premises. He was given some remedies to detoxify his system, an anti-allergen, as well as dietary instructions. I also told him a little story to encourage him.

At a clinic where I once worked we had an organic nursery, from where those patients who were interested were given the opportunity to buy our fresh produce. The experiment was certainly successful and therefore it has been repeated at our clinic in Scotland. One day as I was walking past the nursery, I watched an elderly lady carefully selecting two lettuces. I couldn't help noticing that one of the lettuces showed signs that a slug had spotted the lettuce first. I pointed this out to her and suggested that she might prefer to take another lettuce instead. Indignantly she looked at me and announced, "If it is good enough for a slug, then it will certainly be good enough for me!"

This seems to me to be a very wise observation, because if chemicals had been used a slug would not have been very keen to make a meal of it!

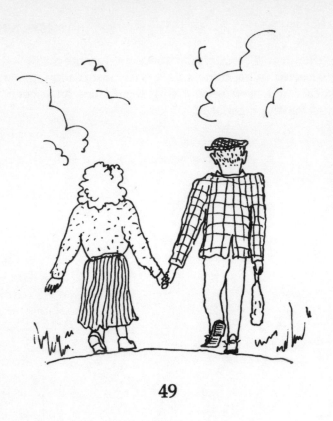

49

Great Expectations

IT JUST SO happened that two of my assistants were at
the reception desk at the same time in discussion with
our receptionist. I was busy in the treatment-room and
needed the help of one of my assistants and so I put my
head round the door to draw the attention of either one
of them. It was then that I witnessed a most extraordinary
scene.

A middle-aged couple were standing in front of the desk
remonstrating with the receptionist that, although they had
not made an appointment, it was important that they saw
the doctor. My receptionist reiterated that any consulta-

tions were only by apppointment and that, in fairness to other patients, it was impossible to bend this rule.

They formed a very odd couple indeed. The gentleman just stood there docilely, barely concealing his admiration for his partner. For all that she was now somewhat annoyed, she too appeared to be a rather timid person by nature. I would have put them both in the late forties to early fifties age bracket and their dress sense was certainly rather unusual. However, one should never judge by appearances.

The lady was now looking decidedly flustered and argued with the receptionist that she just *had* to see the doctor because the matter was urgent and no time was to be wasted. She turned to one of my assistants standing there and pleaded with her to put in a good word for them with the doctor. In response to this most unusual persistence, my assistant said that it was unlikely that an exception would be made, but could she please tell her exactly what she wanted to see the doctor about.

The poor lady's answer floored just about everyone who was within earshot. I quickly withdrew to the treatment-room as I did not trust my reaction if my staff were to spot me. Quite innocently, I am sure, the lady had said, "We've been married more than a week now and I'm not yet pregnant!"

The general titter in the waiting-room was very infectious and when I finally ventured out of the treatment-room, I did not dare approach the desk. Surreptitiously I motioned to my receptionist who followed me into an ante-room and I told her that I would see the persistent couple before I broke off for lunch.

Unfortunately, I discovered when I spoke with them that this rather simple-minded couple had little sense of reality. They told me that they wanted to be like everyone else and have children. I pointed out to them that not every couple had a family and that lots of adults remained childless by choice. They would be able to enjoy their freedom and without the responsibility of children they might get more satisfaction out of each other's company. This was an angle they had never considered before. They left the surgery quite happily and I watched them walk hand-in-hand down the drive.

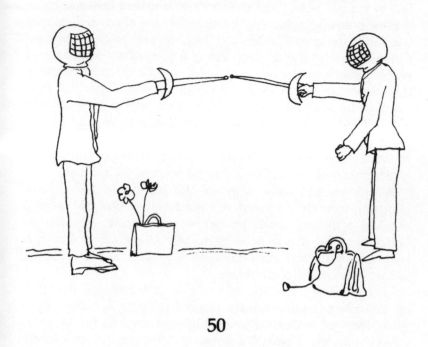

50

A Change of Heart

DO WE OFTEN enough contemplate the contradictory
behaviour of human beings? Mostly we tend to take eccentricity at face value and rarely bother to investigate further
for any possible reasons that lie at the root of it. I know
that it would be a boring existence if we all sported the
same beliefs and opinions, because this would not allow
for any individuality. The resulting predictability of our
fellows would not interest us for very long. However, on
the other hand, I also find it difficult to understand why
some people are so set in their ways that they fail to see

alternative approaches to life. This is a common attitude towards naturopathic or alternative medicine and I would like to tell you about just one such example of obstinacy.

One evening, returning from a lecture abroad, I caught the last flight from London to Glasgow, and bumped into an acquaintance at the airport. He is a journalist, with special responsibility in the medical field and he often appears in interviews on radio and television in that capacity. That evening he seemed very dejected and, trying to snap him out of this mood, I joked with him that it took much more effort to frown than to smile. In order to frown seventy-two muscles have to be activated, while smiling takes only fourteen muscles. That ought to have cheered him up.

We sat next to each other on the plane and he told me about an interview he had recorded earlier that day with a medical professor, with whom we were both acquainted. Unfortunately, this man is extremely dogmatic in his outlook and lacks any conviction that problems can often be solved in more than one way.

This professor has never made a secret of the fact that he considers it unnecessary to give patients a choice as to what form of treatment they might prefer. As far as he is concerned, any form of alternative treatment is absolutely out of bounds. Most certainly he is fierce in his attacks and offensive and rude to whoever dares to disagree with him.

I certainly felt for my friend when he told me about how the interview had progressed; he had been cut short in his remonstrations by this professor every time he raised a point. Little did I know that worse was yet to come.

The following morning, as I waded through the mail that had piled up in my absence, I discovered that I had been selected by one of the medical associations of which I am a member to act as their spokesman at a debate on the benefits of alternative medicine over orthodox medicine. Unfortunately, the other side would be represented by the professor my friend had had the dubious pleasure of interviewing the previous day.

I will not go into detail about our "confrontation", but

most people would have been daunted by his unfriendly attitude, which was clearly apparent even before the debate. I admit that I was rather uptight about the prospect of having to fence with him, but decided that it was time to take off the gloves. I would give him as good as he gave!

He tackled me about unsubstantiated claims on the part of alternative practitioners and the fact that they never seemed to be able to produce any figures or statistics to back up the supposed success of any new form of treatment. I responded by saying that considering the vast amounts of money that were granted to orthodox medicine for the purpose of research, too much of it was spent on producing statistics. I maintained that at all times patients deserved to be considered as human beings, rather than statistics.

I, in turn, raised the subject of the continuous claims of shortages of hospital beds and said that I often wondered just how many of these beds were occupied needlessly. Whatever his or my views were on orthodox, preventive or alternative medicine, I firmly believe that there are fields in which one or other of these approaches excels. Would it not, therefore, be much better if we tried to bridge the gap and concentrated on co-operation?

I must admit that I was rather taken aback when at the end of the debate the professor reached across to shake my hand and stated that I had made some very valuable points and that he accepted them in good grace. I cannot claim that he has now become an advocate for alternative medicine, but he has definitely shed his former blinkered attitude. We have since developed a mutual appreciation of each other's beliefs.

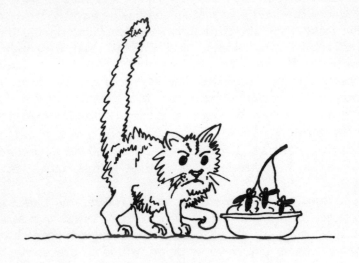

51

A Panacea

I WAS RECENTLY reminded of an unusual case when swapping stories with a good friend and colleague of mine from the Netherlands. While compiling this collection of anecdotes, it sometimes only needed a random remark to bring back to mind a particular case which perhaps had brought to light some unusual aspects of my experience.

My friend and I were discussing a case of epilepsy, when I remembered a lady who had come to the clinic with her young daughter to seek my advice about the little one's bed-wetting. It became apparent that the youngster suffered from a mild form of epilepsy, i.e. "petit mal". The most well-known form of epilepsy is the "grand mal" and I well understand that it is a rather frightening experience for any bystanders who witness such an attack for the first time. A "grand mal" attack will take place without prior warning and the subject will go completely rigid, stop breathing and turn blue. Sometimes he or she will lose consciousness and possibly even foam at the mouth and go into convulsions. After approximately one minute the convulsions will stop and the subject will start breathing again, regain consciousness and after a brief rest will be able to continue with whatever they were doing.

A "petit mal" attack is also often called an "absence" and this latter description is particularly apt for such an attack. These attacks are most commonly experienced by young children and are best seen as a short period in which the subject stares unseeingly ahead and is completely unaware of what is taking place around him. However, with "petit mal" there is no question of losing consciousness.

Nowadays epilepsy can be treated very successfully. Drugs are available to control the convulsions and the major difficulty is that of ascertaining the required strength of the drugs for each individual case, a process which is mostly a matter of trial and error.

A conservative estimate is that one in every two hundred people suffers from epilepsy in one form or another, so it is very likely that someone at your place of work or school, or from your social circle, suffers from this affliction without you even knowing about it.

This particular young girl who was brought to me by her mother seemed to be prone to the milder version of epilepsy, hence her incontinence. It was not deemed necessary to prescribe the usual drugs for her, but I advised that the mother gave her a remedy called Viscum Album, consisting of mistletoe extract. Indeed, she responded well and the "petit mal" symptoms did not reoccur, nor, fortunately, did the incontinence problem.

The mother informed me of this and was obviously very

pleased with the outcome. Then she told me that she could do with my services for herself. Hesitantly, she remarked that she had a few problems herself at night time. She mentioned "hot flushes", but she did not appear to be of the age group that one would automatically assume that this problem was related to the menopause. Eventually, she owned up that she too occasionally found her bed wet and she wondered if the remedy I had so successfully prescribed for her daughter could also solve her problems. I advised her accordingly and she made an appointment to come back to see me again in two months' time.

On her return to the clinic she indeed looked happy enough. I enquired how she had got on and she proudly told me that the remedy had done the trick and that there had not been any further bed-wetting. However, there was just that little something in her manner that worried me. Instinctively, I felt that she was hiding something from me. I had the strong feeling that she had not used the remedy I had prescribed for her at all. I asked her to tell me straight whether she had used the remedy or not. With a mischievous smile she glanced at her husband, who had accompanied her, and he nodded as if to encourage her.

"I am sorry, doctor, that I have not been completely honest with you from the start. Looking back now, I think you may have understood. You see, the cat always sleeps with us in our bed and she has kidney problems. Therefore it wasn't me who suffered from incontinence, but the cat. I thought, however, that you might not want to waste your time on a cat, so I asked you for instructions and then applied these to the cat. Yes, you are right — I did not take the remedy, but I gave it to the cat. And the remedy worked equally well for her, as your prescription did for our daughter. So, the whole family is now indebted to you, including the cat!"

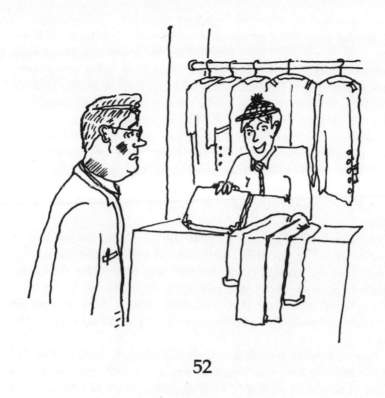

52

A Game of Doubles

MY PARTNER AND influential teacher, Dr Alfred Vogel, had been invited to speak at a gathering and subsequently he asked me to act as his interpreter. This was the usual course of events when he had to speak to an international gathering, because he prefers to speak in his own language — Swiss German. This is not a particularly enviable task, but fortunately I have attended so many of his lectures that I am familiar with his subject and expressions.

I collected Dr Vogel from the airport and we made our way direct to the assembly hall where we discussed

153

the contents of his talk. Going through his material, I promised him that as usual I would do my best to keep up with him and reminded him that we could always imitate Albert Einstein and his chauffeur. The story goes that when Albert Einstein gave his last lecture at the famous Science Institute in New York, he confided to his chauffeur that he hardly felt up to it. His chauffeur came up with an excellent suggestion that rather appealed to Einstein. The chauffeur pointed out that they were of similar stature, both had white hair and a white moustache and, moreover, he had been in the audience so often when Einstein delivered his lecture, that he virtually knew it by heart.

Einstein was delighted to give the go-ahead for his chauffeur to stand in for him, and indeed the lecture went very well. That is, until it came to question time. The chauffeur battled through, but was not able to think of an answer when a member of the audience asked him a specific question. Would the pretence be discovered so late in the day?

The chauffeur handled it ingeniously. He looked blankly at the person who had caused him this headache, shook his head slowly and added, "That question does not speak well for your intellect, because even my chauffeur can give you the answer to that," and pointed to Albert Einstein sitting in the audience.

Dr Vogel and I decided that this role-reversal might work in our case as well, as both of us are short and neither of us has English as our mother language. Moreover, Dr Vogel often used to refer to me as his jack-of-all-trades, because I was his pupil in earlier years, and since then I have acted as his driver, interpreter and often his mouthpiece. The biggest problem was the rather considerable difference in age between us. We checked that no mention had been made in the publicity write-up for the meeting, so we considered that we just might get away with it.

Indeed, I carried it off without even having to resort to the ruse Einstein's chauffeur had been forced to use. At the end of the evening I light-heartedly made my way to the cloakroom to collect our coats and Dr Vogel's luggage, which had been deposited there for safe-keeping.

Much to my surprise, I heard the cloakroom attendant enquire what part of Ayrshire I came from. Just imagine, I had stood on the podium trying to impersonate a Swiss person, and this gentleman in the space of a few seconds recognised my accent and pinpointed it even to the exact county. He told me that he came from Irvine, which is less than ten miles away from Troon where my clinic is situated.

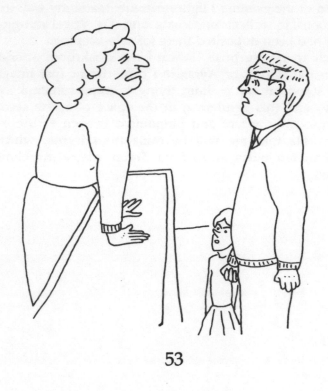

53

Her Heart's Desire

IN THE EARLY days of my practice in Scotland the clinic
was not as time-consuming as it has become in later years,
and it was a welcome break from the extremely busy practice I belonged to in the Netherlands. For various reasons,
it had been quite some time since we had been able to have
a family holiday and therefore we made plans for all of us to
spend a few days in York. It was something we all looked
forward to immensely, as it was indeed a rare opportunity
to spend some time away together.

Since our arrival in Scotland, my young daughter had

struck up a firm friendship with our neighbour's daughter and she had confided in me that she very much wanted a doll like her friend's. In a weak moment I promised her that while we were on holiday, we would see if we could find her one. She then stipulated that it was not just *any* doll she wanted, but it had to be a "doll with a willy". Fair enough, we would see to it.

Later, I wished that I had asked my wife to help, but my daughter made it clear that she quite enjoyed sharing a secret with me and you know what fathers and daughters are supposed to be like, so this father felt rather flattered. The day after our arrival the two of us set off in search of this very special doll.

First of all we went to the toy department of a department store and looked around, but failed to find what my daughter had in mind. I honestly didn't know what she was looking for, but she told me that it was not on show. We went up to the counter and I asked the sales assistant if she could help us as we were looking for a "doll with a willy". First of all the lady looked horrified at me and then told me laughingly that they had no such thing in stock.

We made our way to a specialised toy shop across the road and there we had a repeat performance. Behind the counter were three ladies serving and when I approached one with the request for a "doll with a willy", all three ladies laughed hesitantly and shook their heads. I turned to my daughter and asked her if she was sure that that was what she wanted and uncompromisingly she told me that that was the only doll she wanted.

We left the premises and I told my daughter that we would have one last try and walked towards the market. If we couldn't find what we were looking for there, she would have to go without or we'd ask her mother to look for it in the shops back home.

At the market there were plenty of toys and we looked for the stall with the biggest selection. About half-a-dozen people were serving and there were many customers. Because of the distance between customers and stallholders and the general background noise, I had to raise my voice and called, "Have you got a dolly with a willy?"

A look of disbelief crossed the assistant's face and she asked me to repeat myself. In an even louder voice I asked again, "Have you got a dolly with a willy?"

The general outburst of laughter with which this was greeted was incredible, but still I stood there as I had promised my daughter that this was her last chance. The lady who had been attending to me, looked at me condescendingly and shouted, "Who's next?"

Useful Addresses

Bioforce (UK) Ltd
South Nelson Industrial Estate
Cramlington
Northumberland
NE23 9HL

Tel: (0670) 736537

Nature's Best Health Products Ltd
PO Box 1
1 Lamberts Road
Tunbridge Wells
TN2 3EQ

Tel: (0892) 34143

Auchenkyle
Southwoods Road
Troon
Ayrshire
Scotland
KA10 7EL

Tel: (0292) 311414